ABOUT
FACE

ABOUT
FACE

THE SMART WOMAN'S GUIDE TO BEAUTY

AISLING MCDERMOTT

WITH LAURA KENNEDY

GILL & MACMILLAN

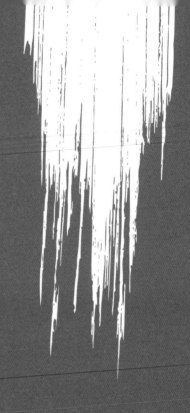

GILL & MACMILLAN
Hume Avenue, Park West, Dublin 12
www.gillmacmillanbooks.ie

© Aisling McDermott and Laura Kennedy 2015

978 07171 6235 2

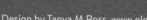

Design by Tanya M Ross, www.elementinc.ie
Photography by Nathalie Marquez Courtney
Styling by Kate O'Dowd
Indexed by Adam Pozner
Printed by Printer Trento Srl, Italy
All photographs supplied by Natalie Marquez Courtney except page 107 (© iStock).

This book is typeset in Brandon Text Light 11pt on 13pt.
The paper used in this book comes from the wood pulp of managed forests. For every tree felled, at least one tree is
planted, thereby renewing natural resources.

A CIP catalogue record for this book is available from the British Library.

5 4 3 2 1

Foreword

One day as part of my job as an editor in *The Irish Times*, I found myself early one morning (far too early if anyone had bothered to ask me) hosting an event called a Beauty Breakfast. We had invited a group of women into our offices on Tara Street in Dublin to give them miniature croissants and assorted berries and to tell them all about our beauty coverage. We wanted to explain that while the newspaper was clearly the place to come to get chapter and verse on highly charged political issues, searing social commentary and major sporting stories, it was also the place to find out whether that new 'luminous' foundation was actually worth fifty of your hard-earned euro or if that 'state-of-the-art' liquid eyeliner was up to the job. The reason I could tell my audience this with such confidence was because hosting the event with me were the two authors of *About Face*, the seriously brilliant *Irish Times* beauty gurus Aisling McDermott and Laura Kennedy.

After I'd done my introduction – during which I laboured a point that will hardly be news to you: that beauty products are hugely important in the lives of many women and, indeed, some men – I let Aisling and Laura do their thing. And they did. A room-full of women asked questions on everything from primers to lipglosses, BB creams to eyebrow pencils while Aisling and Laura provided answers, made suggestions, threw out tips and demonstrated a few make-up fixes.

Eventually the Beauty Breakfast had to come to an end, but the general feeling in the room afterwards was that we could have stayed there all day learning and laughing about the many ways we like to look after and do up our faces. I hope as you read this book, it feels like you are at an event like this with Aisling and Laura, laughing, learning and most importantly getting tips that will save you time and money on the beauty front. Unlike, say, soccer, lipstick isn't a matter of life and death but the right one can put a spring in your step – which is exactly where Aisling and Laura come in.

Róisín Ingle, Daily Features Editor, *The Irish Times*

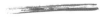

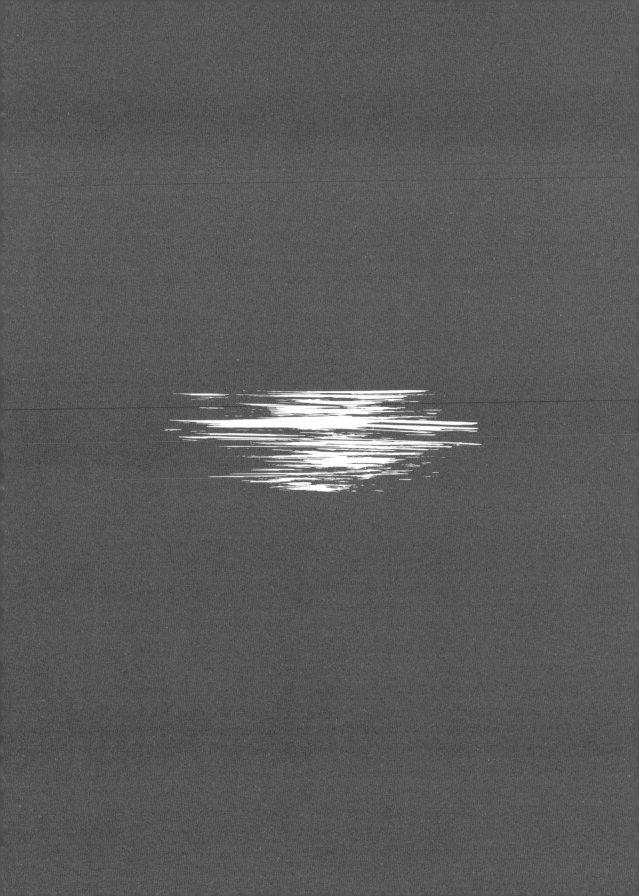

Acknowledgments

We would like to thank our friends, families and the men in our lives for their enduring support and love during the writing of this book. Actually, that makes it sounds like there were lots of men when there were only two. Not two each, two in total. Just one each. As everyone who has ever written a book knows, it's enough to turn you into Bookzilla, so you can appreciate what they had to put up with.

We would also like to thank the fantastic team at Gill & Macmillan for their help, advice and input, which has undoubtedly helped to make this book into something we're very proud of. Thank you to Nicki Howard, Deirdre Nolan, Ruth Mahony, Teresa Daly and Síne Quinn.

Faith O'Grady, the best agent a girl can have, thank you for all your advice and support and for keeping us on track at a time that has been difficult for both of us, for individual reasons. Ditto Róisín Ingle, who also supplied much wisdom and support, definitely deserving of the highest form of thanking possible (i.e. Brandy Alexanders on us).

Thank you also to Orna Mulcahy, Ellen Breen, Nathalie Marquez Courtney and Kate O'Dowd.

Finally, thank you so much to Marian Keyes, Amy Huberman, Panti Bliss, Roz Purcell and Louise McSharry for reading the book pre-publication and giving us such encouraging feedback.

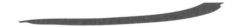

CONTENTS

MAKE-UP

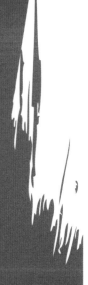

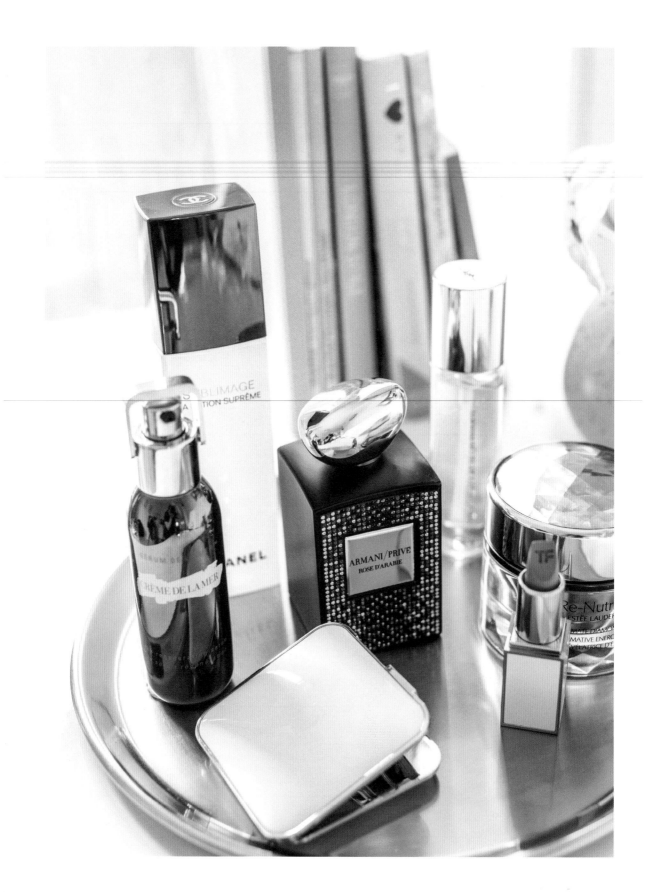

Introduction

've been writing about beauty for quite a long time now and it's pretty safe to say that I've seen lots and lots of beauty trends, fads and products arrive, enjoy their fifteen minutes in the spotlight and move on, to be replaced by the new must-haves and wonder products. The quality of cosmetics, particularly in some of the budget brands, has improved and keeps on improving. Consumers are quite literally dazzled by choice.

Dazzled. Dazed and confused. In a nutshell, that's the reason for *About Face*. There is just so much choice, so much hype and so much jargon thrown around that it is increasingly difficult to know what's good and what's bad, which are the duds and which the diamonds, without spending a whole lot of time and money finding out. We've done the testing for you, narrowed it all down and have done our best to share all our best tips and favourite recommendations with you.

This book is for everyone. Even women who don't think they are 'into' beauty products will always, without fail, have a couple of 'can't live withouts' tucked away. They might not wear make-up but whether it's that one shampoo that can control their hair or the only moisturiser they trust, they'll have something , believe me. And that's all good. A minimal routine with simple, no-nonsense products that work and make you feel good

about yourself means you've got it sorted. Right?

Of course it's right. And then, of course, there is the other extreme – the product junkie. The woman who loves make-up and skincare so much that she devours every beauty website and glossy magazine and subscribes to every Birchbox and Glossybox offering out there. She haunts department store beauty halls and the words 'free sample' make her keel over in a state approaching orgasm. Although she already has over a hundred red lipsticks, there's always room for one (or ten) more. Right?

Yes, also right. Whatever – and I mean whatever – makes you feel good about yourself is what beauty should be all about. Many of us will fall somewhere between these two extremes. If you're reading this book, you probably tend towards the second type but even if you're the first, you'll find some great tips in here.

The problem with the beauty world is that there is an awful lot of deception out there. After almost a decade of writing about beauty, my bullshit detector is set to stun. As soon as I begin to read an improbable press release or look at the ingredients in a massively overpriced vial of serum, I can feel my inner cynic start to snort, like Miss Piggy, in disbelief.

It would help massively if my inner cynic could remain inner at times, but I have no control over her. When sitting in a room surrounded by industry 'insiders' and getting the 'lowdown' on an 'revolutionary' new product that turns out to be a make-up wipe or yet another useless BB cream, my inner Miss Piggy can't help but burst forth. Tossing aside her blonde extensions and rolling her piggy eyes, she often loudly exclaims '*but these things don't work*' and wishes she were at home watching *Keeping Up With the Kardashians* and filing her trotters instead. (As a side note: she also wishes that she was on that show. Naturally they wanted her, but Kim vetoed it. Afraid of the comparisons, you see.)

As you can probably tell, my inner Miss Piggy also has a terrible habit of using air-quotes about just about everything. But I told you – I just can't control her. The fact that she looks like me is also unfortunate, as she is clearly a marketing manager's nightmare made flesh. Miss Piggy hates made-up science – the sciencey-sounding words that the cosmetics industry uses to confuse the bejaysus out of everyone. When she hears that a serum costing €150 is the new 'must-have' (those air-quotes again, sorry about that), she wants to know why. Why is it so expensive? What does it do? If by any unfortunate turn of events she hears that the wonder serum is full of cheap ingredients with only the tiniest bit of the good stuff, she becomes annoyed. Sometimes I can quash her outbursts with a quick internal karate chop but even though others may rave about the newest serum on the block, Miss Piggy actually tests it and knows that it does jack.

See, what Miss Piggy and I both agree on is that we hate being lied to and misled. We hate the deliberate confusion that the cosmetics industry creates in order to push their products and keep their sales and profits high.

Beauty never stands still. It can't. The beauty industry is bigger than the car industry and the fight for market share and innovation is fierce and cut-throat. But while the car industry is tightly regulated – after all, you wouldn't buy a car because 80% of sixty-one men surveyed agreed it went 'quite fast' – the cosmetics industry is not. While a car manufacturer has to stand over every single tiny detail of the cars they build, the cosmetic industry can produce a cream and tell us it will 'luminise', look 'glowy', make skin 'dewy' and could make you 'appear ten years younger'.

Now, how can you test those claims? You can't, because they're meaningless and un-regulated. Lots of words you'll see on labels mean nothing. Hypo-allergenic? You can put that claim on a bottle of bleach if you so wish. Dermatologically tested? Ditto. If someone tells me a car goes from zero to sixty in a certain number of seconds, I can get into the car and find out. It's quantitative, it's measurable.

If someone tells me that a foundation will make me 'appear more youthful', how do I test that claim? It is qualitative – it's a matter of perception and can't be measured accurately. If someone tells me that a peptide will increase the collagen production in my skin how do I test that? I can't. (It won't by the way, but we'll get to that later.)

Most tests that skincare companies quote are done 'in vivo'. This means that someone squirted a concentrated amount of the ingredient onto some cells in a petri dish and a reaction happened. This is where all the misleading sciencey-sounding information about things such as peptides, for example, comes from. In the petri dish the peptides probably did all sorts of amazing things, but the way they work on actual human skin in the watered-down amounts that your serum or moisturiser contain cannot replicate this effect.

What women want is the truth. They want a voice they can trust and that's where *About Face* comes in. There are tons of good products out there and there are stand-out brands, and this is where I start to get excited. There have been vast improvements in skincare in the last few years and it has never been easier to get good skin, to find the right foundation and to learn how to layer your products to find the right mix for you.

There is no wrong way to do anything. We've made suggestions and recommended hundreds of products that we've tried and tested to help you on your way. I have been very lucky to have been joined by Laura Kennedy in the writing of this book – we are different ages, with different skin types, colouring, tastes and experiences in the beauty world. That we are both beauty writers and unashamed product junkies seals the deal. I think our combined expertise has helped to make this book the very best source of information available.

Oh, and yes – one last thing. Foundation is definitely not a feminist issue. Wear make-up or don't wear make-up, it doesn't matter at all. Just enjoy!

Aisling McDermott, 2015

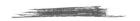

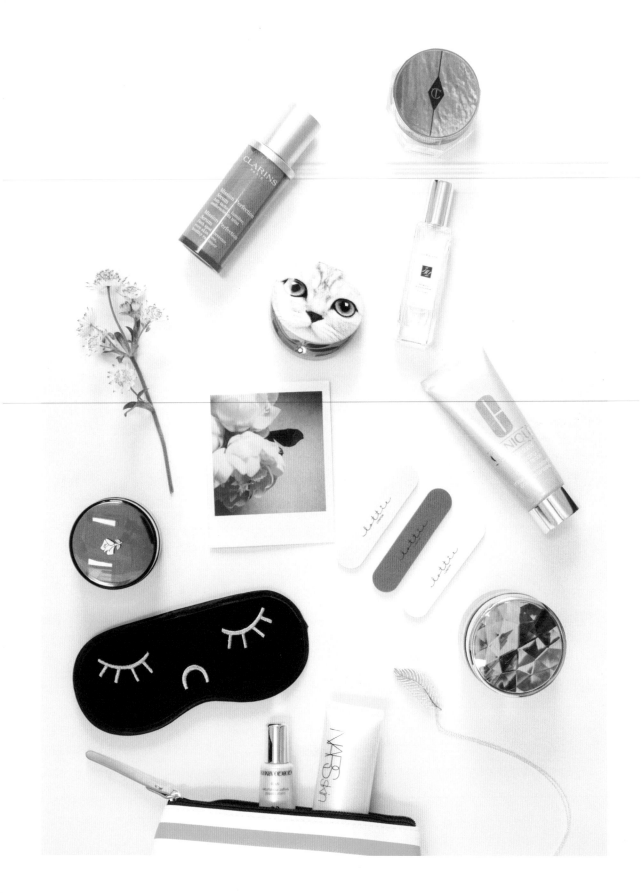

SKINCARE

SKINCARE • CLEANSER • TONER • SERUM • MOISTURISER
• FACIAL OIL · SPF · SKIN CHALLENGES • NECK •

CHAPTER 1

· SKINCARE ·

Before Aisling was born, her Dad worked for Ponds. Yes, Cold Cream Ponds. Because of this, he considers himself an expert in skincare, even though he has had no involvement with the industry for over fifty years. Fifty years, people. And yet conversations with him about the skincare industry often go something like this.

Dad (chortling): *'Grease. Emollients and foaming agents in nice jars. That's all that stuff is.'*

Aisling: *'Yes, once, but now things have moved on and –'*

Dad: *'Ah there's no talking to you women.'*

Aisling: *'Dad, but you worked in the FINANCE department. And this was in the '60s. Surely you must accept that things have moved on quite a bit in the intervening HALF A CENTURY?'*

Dad: *'Nope. But I'll grant you they've probably put a bit more perfume in there or something.'*

So that usually ends that little father–daughter conversation, so they return to talking about their shared love of big German cars or some other neutral topic.

Her father will never fully accept that even though the humble Ponds Cold Cream and Vaseline brands he worked on, which are still around and do remain unchanged, have now been supplemented with some serious skincare. Those traditional favourites are now part of the huge Unilever empire who own tons of other brands – Ren, Murad, Kate Somerville, Dermalogica and Dove, all of whom use new technology and ingredients.

Although there is much phoney science around there have also been some really amazing developments in skincare since Aisling's dad worked in the industry. The widespread use of face-friendly acids, such as hyaluronic, salicylic and lactic acids, together with a deeper understanding of how skin interacts with vitamin derivatives such as retinol, means that skincare these days really rocks.

It is no longer a matter of slapping a bit of cold cream on your face, taking it off with eye-watering astringent toner and hoping for the best. Nowadays, we really understand the importance of sunscreen – the sun is responsible for a whopping 80% of premature skin ageing. With modern skincare products, we can now get rid of sun spots and plump up skin using moisture-attracting oils and serums. Using the right products, we can regulate oily skin and calm down acne and rosacea.

Things really have changed. Layering is a big thing in skincare now – using a handful of different products in the right order each night and morning will make a tremendous difference to your skin. And the developments in serums, liquid exfoliants (also called chemical toners) and many other concentrated sources of skin goodness can help you to have the best skin you've ever had.

Improving your skin gives you a tremendous confidence boost. And that's something not even Aisling's dad would argue with. Or actually knowing him, he might. But he's easily distracted by the sight of a passing new reg Audi so we'll let him off the hook.

The four key skin types and how to tell which you are

No discussion of skincare can begin without identifying your skin type, and it is generally accepted that there are four main categories: normal, oily, dry and combination.

It's easy to find your skin type. Wash your face, do not apply any moisturiser or other products and wait for an hour or two to see how it feels.

Normal skin will feel and look comfortable with no feeling of tightness or oiliness. Your skin is damn near perfect, and no one will tell you this to your face but they secretly hate you.

Oily skin will be shiny and can look greasy straight away depending on how oily you are. Your skin is prone to breakouts, large pores, blackheads and foundation sliding off your face within a couple of hours. Blotting paper is probably your best friend.

Dry skin will feel tight and uncomfortable and if you can last twenty minutes without product, never mind two hours, it will be screaming out for something moisturising to be applied. If your skin is really dry, you'll feel this sensation almost immediately after washing your face.

If your skin tends towards **combination**, you will probably feel a mixture of all of these effects. While your cheeks might feel tight and dry, your nose is often shiny and your chin and forehead aren't be far behind. A lot of us probably fall into the combination category to some degree. The t-zone area (your chin, nose and forehead) can often be oiler and more congested than your cheeks, so taking a targeted approach with your skincare routine can help to even out skin texture. Try using

mild cleansers that won't irritate drier areas of your face and then follow with different treatments on the congested areas to clear them as needed.

However, we actually think it's a bit lazy to categorise skin purely on this basis. The amount of permutations and combinations that exist mean that every single person has different skin concerns existing in tandem. That means there is no neat four-step approach to treating skin types. If there was, this would be a very short book indeed.

Congested skin (the type with blocked pores and lumps and bumps under the surface) exists in both oily and dry skin. Dehydration is the scourge of dry skin – but it also can be the bane of oily skin types, even though they may not realise it. Acne attacks skin at all ages, but particularly during the hormonal hotspots of puberty, pregnancy, perimenopause and menopause. The last two also see a marked decrease in skin elasticity and cell turnover, which leads to lines and less face firmness. And it's no exaggeration to say that rosacea and sensitive skin can make life a misery for those who suffer from these conditions, so they need special treatment too.

To further complicate matters, skin types cannot be categorised without taking age into account. There are four (very general) age categories – all driven by hormonal change – we can identify based on our own observations, through reading literature on and research studies about skincare and make-up, and from years of discussing skin and cosmetics with hundreds of women.

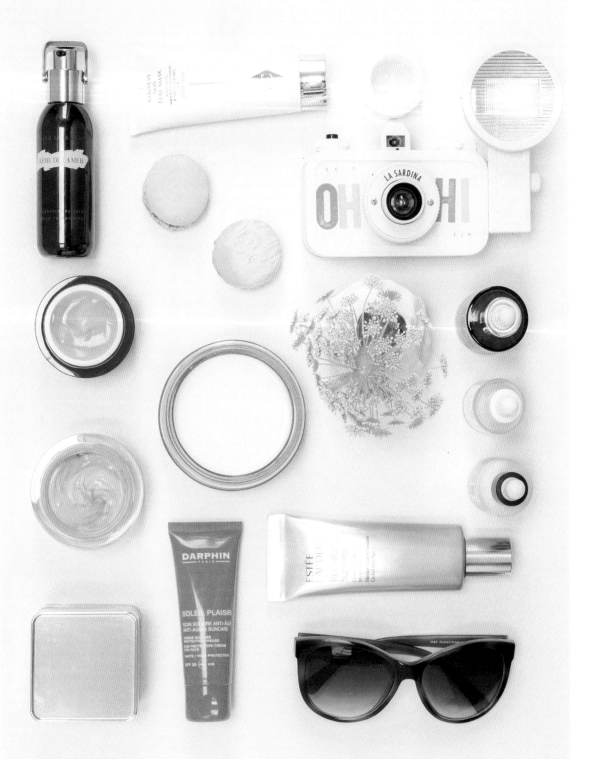

The first is the teen phase, during which hormones send your skin nuts and cause all sorts of spotty, acne and oil-related problems. The second phase is the period that, for argument's sake, we'll say lasts from around the early twenties to the mid-thirties when, illness and hormonal disruption aside, skin should be relatively stable. The third stage tends to hit around the age of thirty-five when skin becomes drier. The fourth is the mature phase, usually from forty onwards, when skin begins to thin and lose elasticity, cell turnover decreases and a load of other things happen that sound dire but they really aren't – they're just a natural part of life.

However, bear in mind that none of this, not one shred of it, is set in stone, and your skin can decide to react and break out at any age – or behave like an angel, just when you are expecting the worst. Some women have skin at sixty that a woman in her forties would be jealous of. And if you are a smoker or suffer from sun damage, you're going to have a completely different experience to a woman who treated her skin well her whole life. Illness also has an impact on your skin, particularly through the use of drugs (prescription or not), and so too, while it has a much smaller role to play than you might imagine, does genetics.

You must treat the skin you have, not the skin you think you should have, and pay little attention to product labelling that tries to herd you into buying products that you may not need. If one of the most beautiful women in the world, Joanna Lumley, finds that Astral Cream works for her in her late sixties and feels no need to 'step up' her routine and use expensive products, then you should take this as a very good example of sticking with what works.

We've got you covered. We've tested hundreds and hundreds of skincare products and now we're ready to share our findings and our tried and trusted routines with you.

Treat the skin you have,
not the skin you think you should have.

The essential skincare routine

Layering products is most definitely a thing in the Western cosmetics sphere at the moment. In days of yore, Western women were content to cleanse, tone and moisturise. In fact, many of us were content just to cleanse and moisturise. A two- or three-step routine suited us just grand.

So what's happened?

One, there are a lot more choices. Remember, once there was only cold cream to take off your make-up. Now the different types of cleanser available run into the dozens. The cosmetics industry rushes in to fill gaps in the market by offering us products we didn't know we needed (and, in many cases, still don't need) and when they sense our interest starting to flag and sales figures go down, they decide to expand existing lines by, for instance, 'going green' and adding a completely new range to their existing offerings.

'Going green' was perhaps the most cynical cosmetics marketing exercise ever, rivalled only by the introduction of Alphabet Creams (see page 143). In the late noughties, every major cosmetic line decided to go 'natural' and 'paraben-free' and embarked upon a ridiculous scaremongering exercise that frightened the life out of people who thought they would harm themselves by using cosmetics containing parabens. But there is absolutely nothing wrong with parabens. They will not harm you in any way – they are a mild-mannered preservative safe enough to be found in many of the foods you eat. However, the cosmetics industry turned their presence into one of evil and fear with absolutely no evidence to support this. And funnily enough, all these green and natural ranges from the big brands just happened, without exception, to cost a fair whack more than the normal lines. Strange that.

This, of course, isn't applicable to the solid 'green' lines that always existed and didn't simply add a 'natural' range to their existing options. Lavera, Weleda, Dr Hauschka and the like are all committed to bringing us natural and organic skincare that is ethically produced.

Two, the internet. The beauty industry has expanded hugely since beauty blogs and vlogs began to offer reviews and show consumers what's out there, how to use it and rave like crazy over the next big thing in cosmetics. Originally not reliant on traditional advertising, unlike magazines, beauty bloggers were free to tell the truth and 'out' the products that were useless. Of course, for every beauty blogger who knows what she's talking about, you'll find three who don't – and unfortunately, not all of tell them tell the truth. But you're intelligent enough to tell the good from the bad and there are plenty of great beauty blogs out there.

Three, layering is what they do in Korea. And by god are we being inspired by Korea like crazy people. Almost all the cosmetic innovation we're seeing at the moment is being copied straight from the massive Asian cosmetics market – see 'Korean Kopying' on page 9 for more. Their routines are bonkers, with ten- to seventeen-step routines common and spending forty minutes in the bathroom of a night is seen as perfectly reasonable.

Really? Forty minutes a night? You must be flaming joking. Let's knock that straight on the head.

No one except extreme skincare junkies is going to go in for those long, elaborate routines. It's not that we're lazy in the West; it's just not part of our culture as it is in Korea. We've taken our skincare cues from the French for so long that to jump from two to twelve steps is far too extreme so five steps are what we propose. Five steps, with the occasional extra step here and there, are manageable, isn't it?

Our essential skincare routine comprises of the following five simple steps. Follow them and, trust us, your skin will improve, congestion will clear up and you'll find yourself using less heavy foundation. This routine can even banish acne and signs of skin ageing. It is suitable for any age and any skin type as all you need to do is tailor your products.

1. Double cleanse

2. Exfoliate

3. Serum

4. Moisturise

5. Oil

See? That's not so bad, is it? Whenever you feel like it, you can add in something extra after the first two steps – a pore-clearing mask, an AHA treatment, a hydrating toner or whatever you feel like doing and you think your skin needs.

However, we do hit a problem with this approach. The big issue is the order in which to layer products. Most people agree that the first three steps are right, but it is the last two steps that have the beauty world all in a lather. It's the seemingly unsolvable beauty equivalent of Fermat's Last Theorem or Schrodinger's Cat.

Some people are adamant that moisturiser should come last because it seals everything in and locks moisture into your skin. And indeed it does, but using it after facial oil also means that the ingredients in your expensive moisturiser don't get a chance to penetrate your skin and might as well be chucked out the window.

Science, on the other hand, tells us that facial oil should come last, after moisturiser, and should be the final thing you put on your face. That's because oil can penetrate moisturiser but moisturiser cannot penetrate oil. However, while this is fine at night, it is definitely not a practical option for the day as oil is a crap base for make-up and will leave your skin looking greasy.

However, we have a third solution. You can quickly solve the entire problem by mixing a couple of drops of oil in with your moisturiser and putting the two of them on your face at the same time.

Bingo. Problem solved.

We've taken our skincare cues from the French for so long that to jump from two to twelve steps is far too extreme. Five steps are what we propose.

Beauty decoded: Korean Kopying

Look to the east. Koreans are simply crazy about make-up and cosmetics. They are not into the serious beauty rigmarole we use here – instead, they love the pure joy and fun of looking after themselves. The packaging of their products is super cute and some of the names they use are hilarious. But just because the packaging might look like something that would appeal to your eight-year-old niece, don't be fooled for a second into thinking the science behind the goods is anything less than world-class.

Many of the new products we've seen in cosmetics lately are either a direct copy of K-Beauty favourites or have been heavily influenced by them; western BB creams, which completely revived the foundation industry and carried it through the recession, are a sad bastardisation of the original and far superior Korean versions. Other K-Beauty innovations making inroads here include cushion foundations, bouncy sleeping masks, waterless foundations, jelly cleansers, sheet masks, snail slime, essences, face shaving and, of course, the rise in multi-step cleansing routines.

But there is one thing that is often overlooked in the rush to uncover the beauty secrets that we're so convinced reside in Korea at the moment. Western brands are just as popular in Korea as their home-grown concoctions, particularly those of the Lauder group, Estée Lauder, Kiehl's, Origins and Clinique.

Another big problem with K-Beauty routines is that they simply just use far too many products all at once. Using three serums, one on top of the other, with only thirty seconds to let each one sink in, doesn't make a bit of sense. The ingredients don't have a chance to work and there's a good chance they may fight against one another and cancel out their individual benefits.

Perhaps the real secret of Korean skincare is their absolute refusal to let the sun near their skin. High-factor sunscreen is only the start. If you have ever travelled in Asia, you will have noticed that many of the girls hold parasols to shield their faces from the sun, wear huge sun hats and plaster stick-on face patches on areas vulnerable to the sun, such as cheeks and noses.

So our real takeaways from the Korean craze should surely be to take our sun protection more seriously and perhaps spend a little longer on our skin routine than before. Notice we're just saying a *little* longer.

CHAPTER 2

· CLEANSER ·

'Cleanliness is next to godliness. But only in an Irish dictionary.'

Yep, this is a famous piece of casual racism that we've all heard a thousand times and it's shrugged off as one of those ridiculous products of another time. But you know what? In a beauty dictionary, cleanliness really *is* next to godliness.

Without proper cleansing, your pores remain blocked and your skin gets rough, dull and clogged with sweat, oil, make-up and just plain old dirt. You're giving bacteria a free pass to romp around on your face creating merry mayhem and breeding spots and blackheads. Oil and dead skin cells remain glued to your skin, sinking into pores and burying themselves until they reach the surface again as a nice unsqueezable whitehead or inflamed pimple. Your skin will look dull at best and it won't matter how much make-up you plaster on. In fact, make-up can just highlight that you're trying to hide bad skin, particularly if you plaster it on thickly to try to counteract the fact that what lurks beneath may not be in great nick.

Cleanser can't change your life. But it can make you feel really confident about your skin and the face you present to the world. Stuff like medication, illness, getting older and skin conditions, such as acne and rosacea, are all things you can't control – but you can absolutely do something about the way they mess up your skin. (We'll talk more about all of that later on.) And doing something all starts with cleansing.

Some of us – most of us – will never have skin that we want to show to the world without any foundation-type product, and we shouldn't feel pressured into thinking that this makes us somehow inferior. It doesn't matter how many ads Cheryl Fernandez Tweedy Cole Versini stars in pretending that a magic blurring product is all you need to look like her. We won't ever look like those women in the ads. And this is without even discussing Photoshop and 'no make-up selfies' in which people quite clearly have half a ton of make-up on and are just posting for the 'U look gr8 hun!' comments.

We're saying a big *kthxbai* to all that crap. Step this way and let us demystify the whole process for you and recommend the cleansing products that really work. Bear in mind that every single one of these cleansers or methods has either been used and approved by us or by someone in our testing pool with the appropriate skin type – and that's the criteria we apply throughout the whole of this book.

You might never have the skin that will make you feel like throwing out your foundation and presenting your naked face to the world, and that's fine. We don't either. But let's talk about how a great cleanser can go a long way to giving you the best skin you can ever have.

Double cleansing

Double cleansing is easy peasy, but the difference it can make to your skin is incredible.

FIRST CLEANSE

Choose a cleanser to remove make-up and surface dirt. This can be anything from micellar water (see page 25) to cleansing oils (Shu Uemura, L'Occitane, Nuxe and L'Oréal all do good ones), creams, balms, jelly and gel cleanser. Just avoid anything that foams. We hate foaming cleansers with a passion and although it's unfair to tar everything with the same brush, so many of them are loaded with alcohol, fragrance and irritating ingredients that it is best to avoid them. Wash your face with your cleanser of choice and rinse with water and a warm facecloth.

SECOND CLEANSE

You may think that your skin is clean at this stage, but we hate to break it to you: it's not. Your first cleanse removed surface dirt and make-up, so now your second cleanse can work to get deep into the pores and dislodge any sneaky grime. For your second cleanse, we recommend a good balm cleanser that you can really work into your skin. This will do the trick: this time when you gently rub off the excess with the facecloth, it will come back sparkling clean.

The best type of cleanser

Cleansers that start out in one form (either as balms or gels), transform into oils when gently rubbed into the skin and then emulsify to a milky mixture when water is applied, are, in our opinion, the best way to cleanse skin when used with a facecloth. The cleanser gently removes every trace of make-up, grime and lime and daily dirt, leaving your face soft and moisturised, while the facecloth does its mild exfoliation thing.

Leave harsh cleansers by the bin or on the shelves unless you've got a specific concern like acne and need a different approach. Switch to balm or gel cleansers and we promise you that your skin will improve – and if you have dehydrated, dull or dry skin it will begin to improve within a very short space of time. There's nothing more satisfying than seeing your make-up turn into a muddy mixture of fifty shades of grey and wash its way down the plughole before you hit the sack. You'll get that experience with these cleansers.

Let's have a look at our top picks. Some of them are expensive, but bear in mind that they will last for ages as you only need a tiny bit each night and when worked out on a cost-per-use basis, they really are worth it.

Clinique Take the Day Off Cleansing Balm is one of the original and best balm-to-oil cleansers. This product has reached cult status and deservedly so. It is quite solid in the tub so you just need to scoop a little bit out and rub it gently into your face. It emulsifies to a milky oil texture and takes everything off. If you are a cosmetics queen and like to use lots of make-up, this is probably one of the

Switch to balm or gel cleansers and we promise you that your skin will improve – and if you have dehydrated, dull or dry skin it will begin to improve within a very short space of time.

best buys you'll ever make as it takes even heavy waterproof make-up off so easily. Clarins Pure Melt Cleansing Gel is a gel cleanser that will dissolve that ten-shade blend of smoky eye very well. Bobbi Brown Extra Balm Rinse is another fantastic balm cleanser, especially for dry skin.

There are quite a few balm- and gel-to-oil cleansers that work very well on oily and combination skin, including Elemis Pro-Collagen Cleansing Balm, The Body Shop Nutriganics Softening Cleansing Gel and Omorovicza Thermal Cleansing Balm. We're beauty-crushing on the whole Omorovicza range at the moment, to be honest, and if you fancy slathering yourself in some jet-black mineral-rich cleanser from Hungary, this mixture will cleanse, draw out impurities and leave your skin spanking clean but still soft. It's good for all skin types but oily, acne-prone and congested skin peeps will love this because it deep cleans without harshness. Black really *is* the new clean.

Oskia Renaissance Cleansing Gel is a bit different because they recommend that you use this pink gel with a dry facecloth – but old habits die hard and we prefer

it with a damp one. As the oil melts, the antioxidants, omegas and pumpkin seeds go to work to exfoliate and reduce irritation and inflammation, making it good for sensitive skin types.

YSL Temps Majeur Cleansing Balm will catapult you into pure luxe skincare territory and is a gel-to-oil cleanser that ticks every box for make-up removal and skin-softening. If you want an ultra-luxurious and moisturising cleanser that nourishes and really pampers skin, then this is the one for you. Aromatherapy Associates Soothing Cleansing Balm is also a lovely balm in a tube that uses calming ingredients like liquorice and camomile to help soothe stressed-out faces.

Beware, though, of the many, many cleansers which are chocca with essential oils. It does make them comforting and with their spa-like smell, tons of people love them. But something full of essential oils is not without its problems as a lot of people simply can't bear the eye watering-ness of this kind of product. If you are sensitive to essential oils, they will sting the eyes off you. In fact, Darphin advise that their Aromatic Cleansing Balm is not suitable

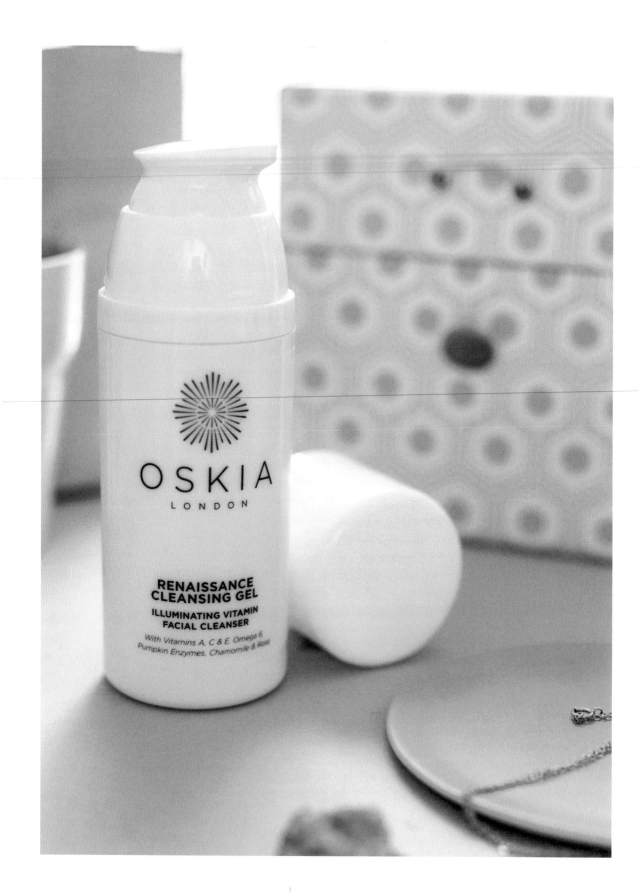

for taking off eye make-up, which is a bit of a pain. Eve Lom's iconic cleansing balm has also fallen slightly out of favour for the same aromatherapy oil reasons (combined with the fact that it contains mineral oil, which is going through a period of extreme unpopularity) but if you're fine with that, aromatic cleansers have zillions of fans and work very well.

Now for the money shot. Emma Hardie Amazing Face Moringa Cleansing Balm has to be our stand-out balm-to-oil cleanser. The mixture is so rich and infused with skin-loving ingredients that it seriously is like giving yourself a facial every night. It's suitable for all skin types, but dry and mature skin will find their skin drinks up this cleanser and thinks to itself 'Where have you been all my life?' Forever more, you will scorn inferior cleansers and it may bring on a panic attack if your tub of oily goodness begins to run out and you haven't reordered in time to instantly replace it with a new one. Don't say we didn't warn you.

Beauty bargain: Budget cleansers

Coconut oil could have been the blueprint for every balm-to-oil cleanser in the world as it is solid in the tub, melts to oil when warmed in the hands and can be easily massaged in to remove make-up, leaving skin feeling incredibly soft. The only problem is that it does not emulsify and dissolve away like commercial cleansers, which means that you will end up with clogged pores. So although we always love a cheap workaround, the downsides of using it as a balm cleanser are too big for us to recommend it as such. As a moisturiser or a night mask though, it's brilliant.

If you are determined to use it as a cleanser, following up with a gentle liquid exfoliator will help to dissolve any traces of the oil on your skin and leave it really clean but still soft.

Another brilliant budget option is Silcock's Base, which will cleanse, emulsify and leave your skin silky soft and clean. A tub costs a few euro, making it a brilliant budget buy and a much better option for your skin's health than coconut oil.

Coconut oil could have been the blueprint for every balm-to-oil cleanser in the world as it is solid in the tub, melts to oil when warmed in the hands and can be easily massaged in to remove make-up, leaving skin feeling incredibly soft.

Cleansing tools

This is one of the greatest cleansing debates: should you use a muslin cloth, a face cloth, a facial cleansing brush or just your fingers when cleansing? Our advice is don't get hung up on the method – there is no right or wrong here.

Facial cleansing brushes like the Clarisonic Skin Cleansing System are the cleansing equivalent of the electronic toothbrush. Dozens of tiny bristles whizz around at lightning speed to unclog pores and leave skin deeply cleansed. They are brilliant for unclogging congested skin and work well with just about any cleanser.

If your skin feels as rough as sandpaper, is oily or blackhead-prone, the Clarisonic or the Clinique Sonic System Purifying Cleansing Brush (which is gentler) will be able to work it all out. Beware, though, that not all of these brushes are created equal: many of them are rubbish, so do your research before you buy or stick to our recommendations. They're also not suitable for every skin type and anyone with skin suffering from an acne flare-up, mature skin or sensitive skin should stick with gentler methods.

Your skin will let you know what feels best and if something feels too rough, then don't use it. Some muslin cloths have the consistency of a Brillo Pad and will irritate delicate or acne-prone skin. Use your fingers if you're going through an intense flare-up; otherwise we recommend a nice soft face cloth used with warm water to gently exfoliate and prep your skin for the next step in your skincare routine.

Actually there is a wrong that we left out. Tissues are pretty rubbish at cleansing and it's best to keep them for blowing your nose.

The best cleanser for each skin type

BEST FOR NORMAL SKIN

People with normal skin are the luckiest – it's already balanced, so you only need to worry about keeping it that way. The world is your oyster – oil, balm, gel or cream cleansers will all be absolutely fine and budget brands will do the job perfectly for you. Go with what makes your skin feel best, but always be suspicious of anything that leaves skin feeling tight or dry after cleansing. And just because your skin is well-behaved, don't take it for granted: alcohol-heavy cleansers can dry your skin out and unbalance it.

BEST FOR OILY AND CONGESTED SKIN

The keyword here is: calm. Calm it all down with soothing cleansers. Oily skin needs to be regulated, so avoid ingredients that are drying. Since it tends to produce more sebum than you'd like, oily skin can be prone to clogging and breakouts, so avoid cream cleansers and alcohol-heavy foaming washes. Laura Mercier Flawless Skin Oil-Free Foaming One-Step Cleanser is a great all-rounder for oily and congested skin while cleansers containing AHAs (alpha hydroxy acids), such as glycolic and lactic acid, and the BHA (beta hydroxy acid) salicylic acid are great for clearing blockages and grimy pores.

A gel, balm or oil formula will make oily skin much happier. Micellar water will work in a fix. And no, oils won't make your skin oilier. We promise.

BEST FOR DRY SKIN

Dry skin is lacking in oil, so the solution is essentially to replace the lost oil in order to soothe and rejuvenate the skin. Begin the process right at the cleansing stage and then continue to nourish with serums, oils, moisturisers and so on. Choose oil, cream or balm cleansers as they will cleanse skin without stripping it, help to replenish lost moisture and balance the skin.

We recommend the following: Yes to Cucumbers Gentle Milk Cleanser, Lancôme Galetée Confort Comforting Milky Cream Cleanser, Nuxe Comforting Cleansing Milk for Face, Eyes and Lips with Rose Petals, Philosophy Purity Made Simple One-Step Facial Cleanser, Trilogy Cream Cleanser, Uriage Crème Lavante Cleansing Cream and Elave Sensitive Rejuvenating Cleansing Treatment.

For great low-cost alternatives, try Nivea Daily Essentials Gentle Cleansing Cream Wash for Dry and Sensitive Skin or Johnson's Daily Essentials Nourishing Cleansing Lotion for Dry Skin.

On the pricier scale, you can't go wrong with Clarins Extra-Comfort Anti-Pollution Cleansing Cream and Clinique Comforting Cream Cleanser.

BEST FOR SENSITIVE SKIN

Sensitive skin needs a cleanser as free as possible from fragrance, additives, scrubby bits and potential irritants. Avoiding fragrance is particularly important as it is the most common reason for reactions. Choose unperfumed lotions and potions as much as possible and bear in mind that just because something is 'natural' it doesn't mean that you won't react.

Have a sniff of something before you buy it. If your immediate reaction is 'Eww, that's a bit strong', this is the first indication that you may react to the product so avoid it – streaming eyes, rashes and hives are no fun.

If you've got sensitive skin, some of the best cleansers are Avène Tolerance Extreme Cleansing Lotion, Cetaphil Gentle Skin Cleanser, Simple Kind to Skin Purifying Cleansing Lotion, Burt's Bees Sensitive Facial Cleanser, The Body Shop Aloe Gentle Facial Wash and Clarins Extra-Comfort Anti-Pollution Cleansing Cream.

BEST FOR ACNE-PRONE SKIN

Adult acne is a scourge and is the most common skin problem in women over forty. The menopause throws skin off just as much as adolescence does, so be guided by what works for an oily skin type. Avoid shea butter and other congesting ingredients and although you might feel like hitting up the Sauvignon Blanc to console yourself, don't even consider using alcohol anywhere near your face.

Essentially, though, the problem is hormonal and skincare will only go so far. Don't be afraid to admit defeat if acne is affecting your self-esteem. See a dermatologist for professional advice if you need to.

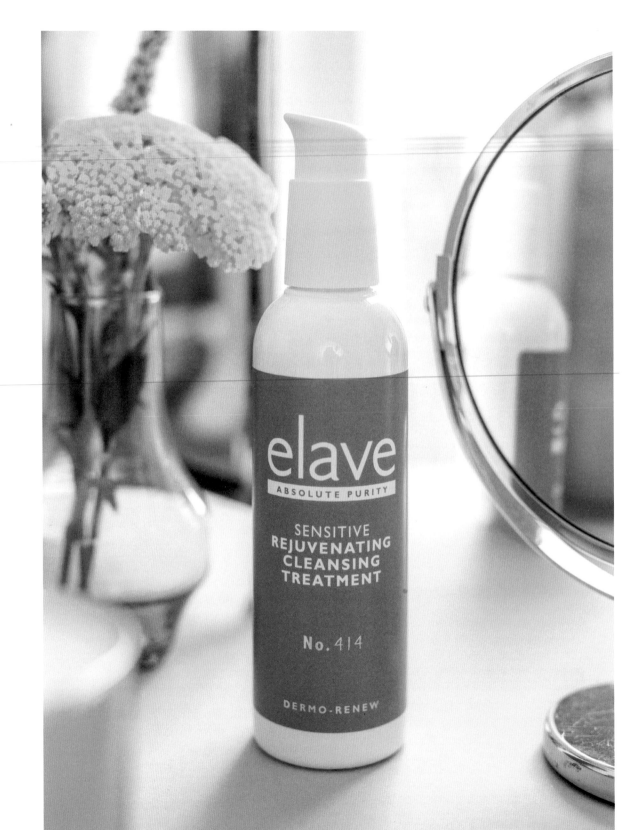

BEST FOR MATURE SKIN

Mature skin needs extra love and nourishment and this has to start at the cleansing stage. Super-rich balm and oil cleansers can only do you good. Ingredients that clog younger skin, such as shea butter, are perfect for injecting moisture into more mature skin, so try L'Occitane Shea Cleansing Oil for a rejuvenating cleanse. A gel-to-oil formula will also get on well with mature skin, but avoid anything drying.

Cleansers with glycolic acid increase cell turnover, which slows in mature skin, plus they unblock pores and reveal fresher, younger skin straightaway. Try Elave Age Delay Daily Cleanser or Jan Marini Bioglycolic Face Cleanser. Just make sure to keep these products away from your eyes – acids and eyes are a bad combo. Also worth trying are NeoStrata Foaming Glycolic Wash and Nip+Fab Glycolic Cleansing Fix, but go easy with these, or avoid altogether, if your skin is fragile. If you find them too harsh, restrict your use to just once a week or substitute with a gentle exfoliating toner after your cleanser, which will essentially do the same job.

BEST FOR TEEN SKIN

Teen skin is undergoing a big transition. It's going to misbehave, so try to tackle issues without feeling too bad about them – if you're suffering with breakouts, you're certainly not alone. Cleansing is very important for teen skin because bacteria levels can be hard to regulate and using the wrong products can drive skin out of control. Just don't, for the love of God, pick a product loaded with astringents or alcohol.

The most important thing is to keep skin balanced. Avoid applying anything laced with alcohol and resist the urge to 'dry out' the dreaded spots. It's tough, but try to let them run their course without picking. Using a soothing oil or balm cleanser twice daily and incorporating a glycolic wash into your routine once a week won't stimulate oil production and will help to prevent scarring. If acne becomes unmanageable, seeing your GP to discuss your options is always a good idea.

Acne can be very tough to deal with and sometimes topical products just aren't enough. Don't suffer with it – it can be sorted, or at least calmed down considerably.

Beauty decoded: Face-friendly acids

ALPHA HYDROXYL ACIDS

Alpha hydroxy acids (AHAs), particularly glycolic and lactic acids, are used to exfoliate, increase cell turnover and diminish the appearance of fine lines. They are particularly effective when used in cleansers and toners. AHAs gently 'unglue' sticky dead skin cells and allow your serums and oils to work properly. Face masks with a good helping of AHAs will clear up skin and are a great pro-ageing ingredient. We're hooked on this ingredient because it quite simply works.

BETA HYDROXYL ACIDS

Beta hydroxy acids (BHAs) are different: there's only one of them – salicylic acid. Salicylic acid is a stand-out ingredient in the treatment of spots, blackheads and areas of congestion. It works by penetrating the hair follicle where blockages start to build up, and controls the amount of bacteria on the skin's surface. It's a brilliant ingredient for teenage and acne-prone skin as it can actually get rid of blackheads and, with regular use, stop pores filling up with oil again. If you use a scrubby scrub to exfoliate, you are only removing the dead cells on the skin's surface; this ingredient goes much further. Use it in cleanser, toner and face creams.

EFAS

Essential fatty acids (EFAs), such as linoleic acid and omegas 3 and 6, are great at reducing inflammation, moisturising and nourishing skin when consumed as part of a skin-friendly diet. They also work in topical skincare so look for them in facial oils, serums and moisturisers where they will have a chance to sit on the skin for the longest possible time. They're good for just about everyone and really come into their own when used for conditions like rosacea. You'll find them in a lot of skincare – look out for compounds like glycerin, sterols and phospholipids in ingredient lists.

HYALURONIC ACID

A humectant with the capability to attract over 1000 times its own weight in water from the air and saturate skin with moisture, it's no wonder that hyaluronic acid is enjoying a moment. It's a sure thing for anyone with dry or dehydrated skin and is great in serums, moisturisers and masks, particularly night or sleeping masks. If you're using it in a serum, seal it in with moisturiser. Although you can get cleansers with this ingredient, they're not going to do much hydrating as the hyaluronic acid will be washed straight off, so it's not really of any benefit in cleansing.

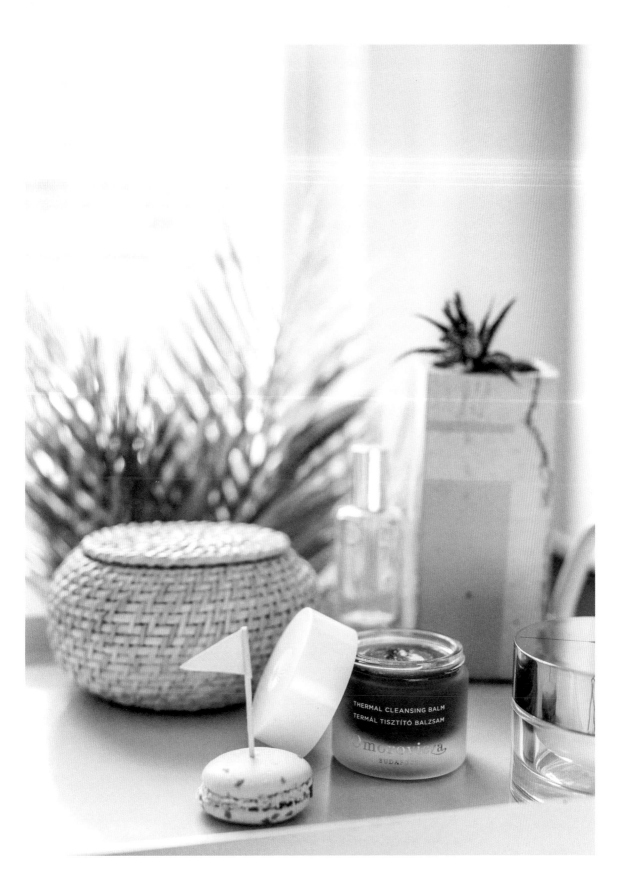

A sticky one this, as a lot of people prefer their products, from cleanser and foundation to lip balm, in a tube or a vial with a pipette, because they think tubs are unhygienic.

There is something to be said for this, as sticking your fingers in a pot of cream day after day contributes to germs and gremlins entering tubs and jars of cleansers and moisturisers. The answer to this is easy: don't let other people use your products and wash your hands before you use them.

We get the concerns, but unless you're sharing with ten other people who have questionable hand-washing practices or applying your lipstick straight from the tester in the chemist, you're probably okay and will not die.

Jars are fine. Don't worry about it too much. Or at all.

Eye make-up remover

If you're using an oil-based or gentle creamy cleanser, then there is no need for a separate eye make-up remover. Just smooth on your regular cleanser until you have a nice black panda-esque eye area and then rinse off (you can use cotton wool if you don't want to use your facecloth). If you've applied a hundred coats of mascara and know they're not going to shift without a fight, soak a cotton pad with cleanser and press it over the eyelashes for a few minutes to soften and dissolve the gunk.

If you're dead-set on a separate remover, pick an oily one to moisturise the eye area and lift off even stubborn waterproof make-up more easily. Clinique Take the Day Off Makeup Remover for Lids, Lashes & Lips is good for heavy waterproof addicts, while Nivea Daily Essentials Double Effect Eye Make-Up Remover is a good budget oily option.

If you want to go with a non-oily version, Lancôme Bi-Facil Non-Oily Instant Eye Makeup Remover has been around forever and is a bestseller for a reason. Other good options are Bourjois Express Eye Makeup Remover and Avène Gentle Eye Make-up Remover.

The use of alcohol in skincare products

Alcohol is used almost universally in skincare products and it's very bad news for skin. It instantly dries it out, producing a temporary feeling of tightness and that 'squeaky clean' feeling. While you may long for this feeling if you have oily skin and equate it with the best way of cleansing, trust us, it is not. Your skin should always feel soft and nourished, no matter how much you long to blast that greasy nose into the stratosphere with the most powerful chemicals this side of the atomic bomb.

Resist the urge to turn to the bottle. Alcohol sucks the moisture out of the upper layers of the skin and the body responds by pulling oil up from deeper down in the dermis to compensate. So although you may think that the bright blue

Beauty decoded: Products containing alcohol

As alcohol is such a widely used ingredient, you may find that some of our product recommendations contain small amounts of it. Sometimes it is necessary to have some in a formula to keep other ingredients stable, particularly those containing AHAs.

To further confuse the life out of us, some ingredients that have alcohol in their name are not alcohol. For example, stearyl alcohol and decyl octyl alcohol are compounds produced from stearic acid, a naturally occurring fatty acid that is moisturising for skin. There are lots of other examples, so unless an ingredient is listed as isopropyl, alcohol or alcohol denat, it's probably fine.

bottle of toner you've splashed all over your face has made it pleasingly matte and sorted out all your problems, it hasn't. It has, in fact, just caused a chain reaction that will make your skin even oilier and more irritated.

Those with dry, sensitive skin and rosacea shouldn't touch products containing alcohol with a bargepole. It will cause you untold misery: stinging, flushing, flaking skin and intense dryness.

Products aimed at the teen market, those who are most concerned with oily skin and breakouts, are usually loaded with alcohol. Look at the ingredients and if the first or second on the list after water (eau) is alcohol, isopropyl or alcohol denat, put it back on the shelf.

If the cleanser is bright blue, that might also be a dead giveaway. #JustSaying

Make-up wipes

Ditch the wipes. Trust us, please trust us. Ireland's bestselling beauty products, outperforming any other cosmetic out there, are make-up wipes. We understand – you're tired and you don't want to wake up with the Shroud of Turin on your pillow. Maybe you've just fallen into bed three sheets to the wind and it's either wipes or nothing. We do it ourselves. But wipes are bad news – they're loaded with alcohol, which dries and irritates skin, and they're simply not wet enough to do anything but push the make-up around your face and take off the barest surface dirt.

In the interests of public safety, we've done the wipe test – under laboratory conditions obviously. Our faces looked cleanish but when we did a proper cleanse afterwards with a hot cloth and decent cleanser, we could see the evidence on the white facecloth we used: it was filthy.

When you're in a hurry, use micellar water or a jelly cleanser. We love this new Korean import and Bio-essence have a lovely fresh, quick cleanser, Miracle Bio Water Jelly Makeup Remover, that's suitable for all skin types.

Face wipes are useless. The end.

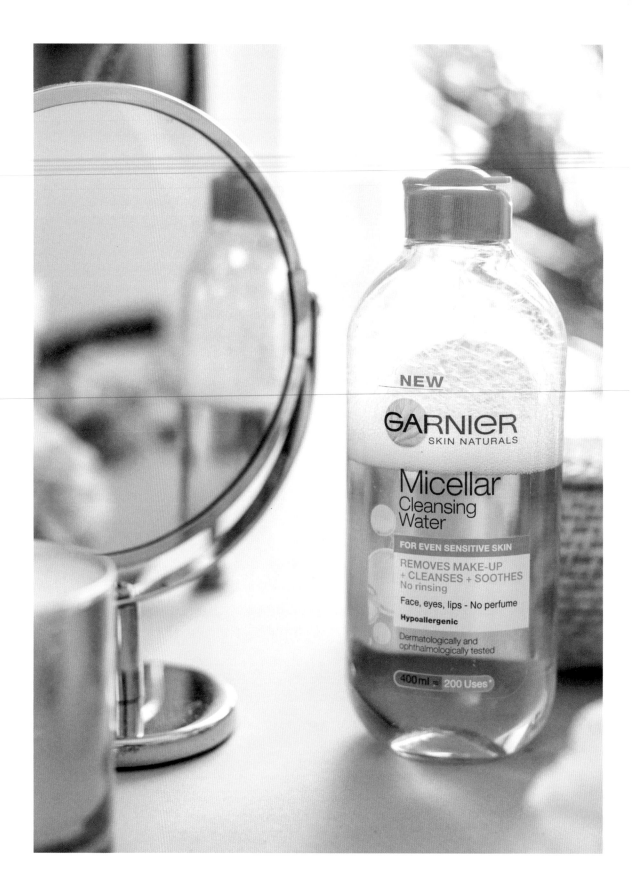

Micellar water

Micellar waters are the new-age answer to lazy girl problems. Micellar water is a sciencey combination of oil and water molecules that cleanses far more efficiently than a wipe ever could and, most importantly, doesn't contain any alcohol to dry the life out of your skin. Swoosh the water on a cotton pad when you can't be bothered to double cleanse and you will remove make-up and surface grime far more efficiently than a wipe ever could. It's also a handy one to keep around as a first cleanse product.

Micellar water will be your lifesaver on those nights when you're so knackered you wish fairies would come and transport you to bed, take off your boots and put on your pyjamas for you. You can even keep a bottle by your bed together with some cotton pads and take off your face while lying in bed. Not that we have ever done that or anything.

Foundation and blush can generally be removed with a couple of swipes unless you're Kim Kardashian, but eyeliner and mascara need a bit more care. To remove heavy eye make-up with micellar water, soak the pad with water and press over your closed eye for a couple of minutes. Don't scrub – just keep patting and pressing until the make-up is removed.

A bottle of micellar water is never a waste of money but it makes no sense to buy an expensive one. Stick with a cheaper brand like Garnier Micellar Cleansing Water, Bioderma Sensibio H2O Make-up Removing Micellar Solution or Boots Botanics All Bright Micellar 3 in 1 Cleansing Solution.

Micellar water will be your lifesaver on those nights when you're so knackered you wish fairies would come and transport you to bed.

CHAPTER 3

· TONER ·

Toner is back in vogue. After years in the skincare wilderness, it has suddenly become wildly popular, with many women adjusting their regimes to add an extra product. How did this happen?

In a word: rebranding. Many products now labelled as toners are actually chemical or liquid exfoliators. These are the good guys and the ones we're going to talk about because we really, really don't rate the other two types of toner. One is actively bad for your skin while the other is not much cop at all.

Toners were invented to cut through the grease of heavy cleansers, but cleansers are now so good that they wash off your face without leaving any residue. However, on the back of the success of acid toners, every product labelled 'toner' has gained in popularity, even the ones that would tear the face off you so read on to discover which ones are worth it.

The three different types of toner

Toners can be loosely divided into three categories.

CLARIFYING/ASTRINGENT TONERS

Astringent toners, the original of the species, haven't changed much since the beginning of time. If you were a glamorous, make-up-loving lady back in the day, then you'd remove your make-up at night with something like cold cream (think of a thick, creamy make-up remover like products from brands such as Ponds, but even heavier). You'd whack a blob of that onto your face, the mineral oil in the cleanser would melt your make-up and you'd tissue off the excess. But your face would be slimy from cleanser. To dissolve the layer of greasy cleanser, so that there was no barrier to the absorption of your subsequent skincare (it was never getting through that layer of oil), you'd need an alcohol-based product. Clarifying or astringent toners are like these old-fashioned toners and they are evil. Basically paint-stripper.

These days, cleansers are more effective and we don't need to dissolve residue after cleansing, so traditional toners are marketed to people with very oily skin and acne. If you suffer with these issues, please don't use these products unless they're prescribed by your dermatologist and you really must. As someone with a long history of acne, Laura can fully appreciate the frustration of clogged, dull, sore, red, bumpy skin that feels smothered by its own oiliness. You just want it to go away, so you try to dry up the oil with alcohol. And alcohol will dry up your oily skin very briefly. But then it will make it much, much worse. The more alcohol you apply to your skin, the more you encourage oil production. You'll end up more acne-prone and oilier but with tight, flaky, painful skin. It's not worth it.

Clarifying or astringent toners are usually loaded with ingredients such as alcohol and witch hazel (a little of this is fine, a lot isn't) and often promise to reduce oil and pore size and to refresh skin. Nothing can make pores smaller, and these ingredients irritate and dry out many people's skin. They're often cynically marketed at teen consumers who are desperate to get rid of spots and blemishes. Traditional toners are simply not worth the money; you're better off investing in a good cleanser.

HYDRATING TONERS

The second type of toner promises to 'hydrate and restore the skin's pH balance' and often claims to contain only 'pure and natural ingredients'. Many beauty experts regard this type of toner as being as useful as pouring your money down the sink, because you can get all the moisturising you need from your serum, oil and moisturiser. Lots of women love these toners though, as they're cooling and refreshing. If you are a fan, choose an inexpensive brand or try simple rosewater.

CHEMICAL / ACID TONERS

Now these are the ones we're interested in because they act as very gentle exfoliators along with other benefits. Read on to find out why they're one of the best things you can treat your skin to.

Choosing your exfoliating toner

Toner is the new exfoliator. Exfoliation doesn't mean what it used to. The days of gritty physical exfoliants and the dreaded peach kernel that would rip the face off you are long gone. A much better way to sweep away dead skin cells and unblock pores is to exfoliate using acid or liquid toners on a cotton pad. Chemical exfoliators dissolve away dead skin using mild concentrations of enzymes or acids. They instantly brighten the complexion and can improve conditions such as acne, which explains why they are so popular.

Gritty physical exfoliants are more trouble than they're worth. We tend to use them too enthusiastically and end up pulling the skin, causing swelling. If your skin is red or hot after exfoliating, you've been too rough. Physical exfoliation can cause broken capillaries (which can only be removed with laser treatment) and can seriously inflame broken or acne-prone skin. Ditch the grit for an AHA toner.

Plus you know those plastic beads in a lot of exfoliators? Hopefully they will be banned before this book is published as they are an environmental hazard: they don't dissolve and end up in lakes, rivers and the sea, choking fish and silting up waterways.

Post-cleanse products or acid toners containing the AHAs glycolic, lactic and salicylic acids have been ingeniously branded to fit into the magical three-step skincare myth of 'cleanse, tone and moisturise'. So when a modern skincare junkie talks about toning, they are usually talking about liquid or chemical exfoliation. Don't be frightened of the terminology. It simply refers to the use of products that contain AHAs such as glycolic acid to increase cell turnover in the skin, keeping it smooth and at the optimum level of absorption for skincare. AHAs are used by dermatologists for chemical peels, but the levels contained in exfoliating or acid toners are very minimal – anything you can buy over the counter is never going to be overly strong. Essentially, AHAs like glycolic acid dissolve the bonds between dull, dead surface skin cells, gently separating them and exposing the fresh new skin underneath.

Exfoliation doesn't mean what it used to. The days of gritty physical exfoliants and the dreaded peach kernel that would rip the face off you are long gone.

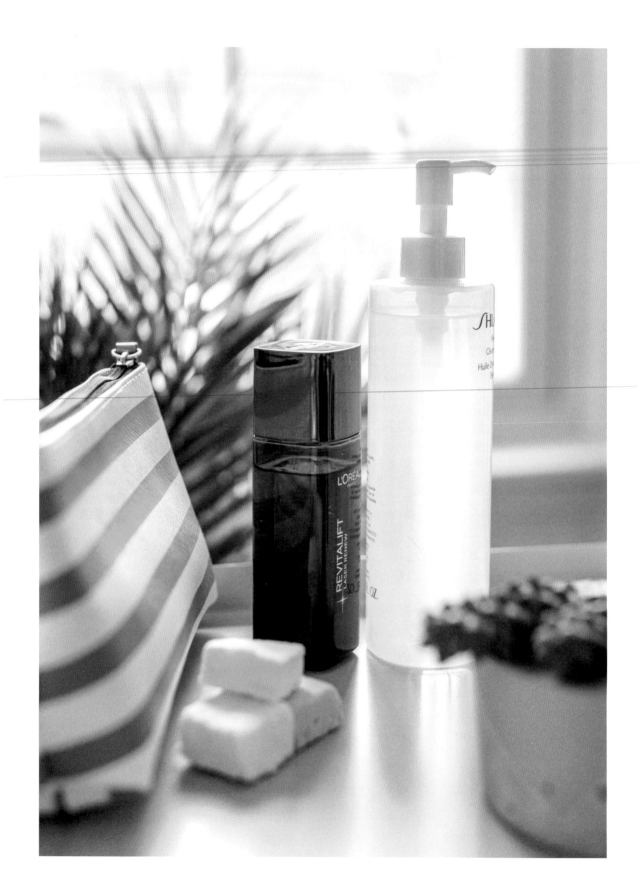

Obviously, you should tailor the AHA percentage in a product to the sensitivity of your skin. The more sensitive or reactive your skin, the lower the percentage of AHAs you should use in your toner. Acid toning is beneficial for any skin type – except hypersensitive skin or for anyone with associated allergies. Glycolic acid is a natural acid you'll find in fruit like strawberries so it's nothing to be afraid of.

There is one essential point to remember when using any product which contains AHAs.

Glycolic acid products make your skin sensitive to sunlight, so you must use a separate SPF. Using a moisturiser that contains SPF is not enough. If you don't use SPF every day while using AHAs, you will prematurely age and genuinely damage your skin. Use them correctly though, and they will keep skin texture smooth, heal mild scarring (the red sort you get from a nasty spot) and help your other skincare products to absorb optimally.

Chemical exfoliators dissolve away dead skin using mild concentrations of enzymes or acids. They instantly brighten the complexion and can improve conditions such as acne.

The best exfoliating toners

Clarins Gentle Exfoliator Brightening Toner is an all-time favourite and can make a fantastic difference to your skin. Use up to twice daily after cleansing. It does contain a small amount of alcohol, which is not ideal, but this is counteracted by some other nice ingredients like glycerine, so it won't dry out your skin.

Aveda Botanical Kinetics Skin Firming/Toning Agent and Alpha H Liquid Gold with Glycolic Acid are also a good investments, as is Pixi Glow, which is a more natural alternative. Pixi Glow contains around 5% glycolic acid, making it more potent than the Clarins equivalent, and combines urea with natural ingredients like witch hazel. Maintaining a healthy pH level on the skin is essential – when skin pH is off, conditions like dermatitis and acne can appear or worsen because bacteria levels on the skin aren't balanced.

L'Oréal Revitalift Laser Renew Peeling Night Lotion, one of Aisling's staple products, is a very effective chemical exfoliating gel with glycolic and lipohydroxy acid that smooths and can help to combat dark spots too.

Mario Badescu Glycolic Acid Toner contains just 2% glycolic acid, so it's suitable for more sensitive skin but will still encourage cell turnover and brighten the skin. It also has soothing aloe to help with sensitivity. Ren Clarifying Toner is the gentlest on the toner list, and so is ideal for very sensitive skin. Rather than the more vigorous glycolic acid, it contains lactic acid, which provides very gentle cell renewal. Again, this one contains some alcohol, but there are other ingredients that compensate for this. If your skin cannot tolerate glycolic acid, then this might be a good option for you.

If you can cope with more potent quantities of glycolic acid, then Paula's Choice Skin Perfecting 8% AHA Gel Exfoliant is one to try. More of an exfoliating mask than a toner, it contains a high concentration of AHAs. You might notice some stinging when you first apply it but it provides very effective exfoliation and is great for oily, congested skin. There's also a generous measure of hyaluronic acid in there, which ensures that your skin will not be left feeling dry. This potency isn't for newbies – only use this on skin which is accustomed to lower percentages of glycolic acid already.

And although it is not a liquid toner, this is the most brilliant product ever and everyone we recommend it to falls instantly in love: Ren Vitamin C Flash Rinse 1 Minute Facial brightens and smooths by removing dead, flaky skin almost instantly. Don't overdo it, though: a couple of times a week is more than enough for amazeball results.

Beauty decoded: Face shaving

It is not only Korean beauty rituals that have gripped the imagination and changed the habits of Western women; recently, another commonly practised Eastern beauty ritual has gained thousands of enthusiastic Western fans. A widespread method of exfoliation in Japan, face shaving has caught on in the West, with women shaving their entire faces from cheeks to chin. We're not among them as we think this is probably one of the worst ideas in skincare but it has been popular in the East for centuries, and with our current passion for all things Asian plenty of Western women are getting on board with it. In fact face shaving is nothing new as women have been shaving for thousands of years, with everyone from Cleopatra to Marilyn Monroe. (Even Elizabeth Taylor is reported to have been partial to whipping out the razor on occasion.)

For years no one knew what Japanese women were doing in the bathroom every morning. Their whole family could have been banging on the bathroom door, late for work and school, but they were busy, beautifying themselves for the day by painstakingly shaving their faces. No, not just the bit that the waxer might have missed above their top lip or that stray chin hair that sprouted in the night – which, everyone knows, only happens when you can't find a tweezers. Japanese women shave their whole faces, including all the downy hair from their cheeks.

So why would anyone want to do this? It seems strange, in a world where there are plenty of other longer lasting hair-removal treatments such as wax, threading, laser and IPL.

Enthusiasts, and there are many, proclaim that the procedure leaves them with softer skin, exfoliates and ensures make-up goes on more smoothly. Now we are not talking about lathering up with a Mach 3 and rasping a five-blade razor across delicate lady skin – specialist, one-blade razors are used to gently trim hair. Brands such as the bestselling Tinkle and Shiseido produce tiny razors very cheaply and a pack of three will set you back less than a fiver on Amazon. However, it is a mistake to think that men's skin ages better than women because of a lifetime of shaving: it is simply because they have thicker, oilier skin, so we can throw that face-shaving 'benefit' out straight away.

Vellus hairs are the fine, light-coloured downy hairs that everyone has on their face. In most cases, they are virtually invisible, but some of us have furrier faces than others and when make-up is applied over these tiny hairs it has the effect of coating them and making them thicker and more visible. The phenomenon of the Foundation Moustache (see page 122) is a direct result of vellus hairs being coated in foundation and then topped with a layer of powder, which makes them stand out proudly in 3D relief.

But before you reach for the razor, bear in mind that the only person your downy facial hair might be visible to is … you.

Beauty decoded: Essences

Essence products are our new skincare favourite and we're dying with excitement over them, as they exfoliate even more gently than toner. Another import from the world of K-Beauty, an essence is a sort of watery serum. Just like serums, different essences will have different skincare benefits depending on their active ingredients – some will brighten, some provide hydration and so on.

Koreans use them after cleansing and toning and before serum – and funnily enough, when researching essences, Aisling realised this is exactly how she's been using Estée Lauder Advanced Night Repair. On nights when her skin is really dry and cranky and she feels that Tutankhamun probably has a fresher complexion than she does, she uses L'Occitane Shea Cleansing Oil with a facecloth to exfoliate. She follows this with Estée Lauder Advanced Night Repair, lets it soak in for a few minutes and then puts a hydrating serum on top (usually whatever is waiting to be tried out for testing purposes), before mixing some facial oil with a rich moisturiser and patting it in.

We realise that this seems like a million steps but this kind of layering is brilliant for dry or tired skin. Grab a cup of tea, a good book and sit up in bed having a relax for twenty minutes so that the whole lot has a chance to sink in.

If you're ready to embrace an essence, Kiehl's Iris Extract Activating Treatment Essence gently clears dead skin cells while hydrating at the same time. Tom Ford Intensive Infusion Treatment Essence is another watery skin-softening option, as is L'Occitane Pivoine Sublime Perfecting Essence. Clinique Even Better Essence Lotion, a mix of antioxidants and anti-irritants, is very good for hydrating and softening dry or combination skin. And hopefully, before too long, even less expensive Western brands will be jumping on the essence band wagon.

Essence products are our new skincare favourite and we're dying with excitement over them, as they exfoliate even more gently than toner.

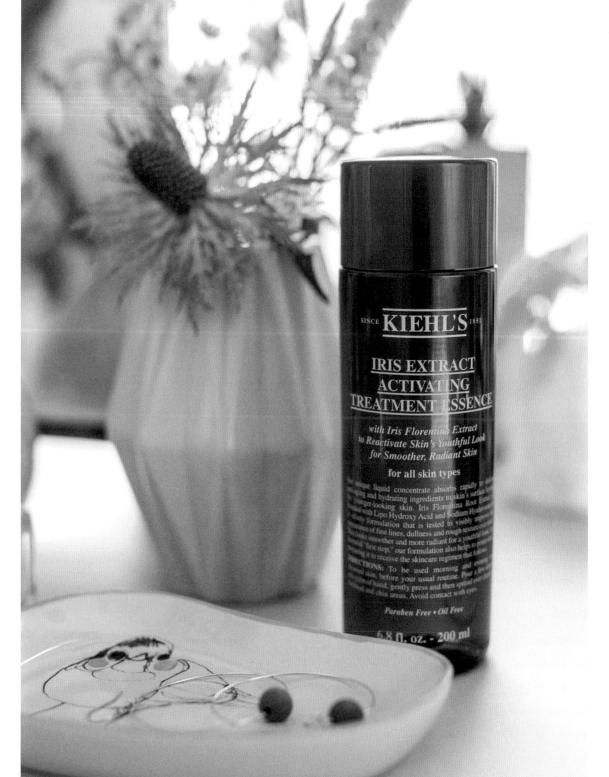

Face masks

Brighten up your skin with a facial. Or maybe not.

If your skin is feeling dull and dreary, sometimes the best way to cheer it up and get it looking like something that belongs to an actual human person is to get a facial. *What better way to brighten up that skin than to book in for a salon facial,* you may say to yourself. *Why only yesterday,* you may think, *I saw a great offer for an hour long facial for only €20. I think I will treat myself,* you promise.

While going for a facial is honestly one of our favourite things in the world to do, you must remember that all facials and all salons are not created equally. Yes, there are great deals on at the moment and so there should be because everything was shockingly overpriced there for a few years – and actually it still is to be honest, but that's a conversation for another day.

While most people find a salon and a therapist they trust and can return to again and again, as beauty writers we are duty bound to try out as many salons and treatments as we can. If we do not know about something, we cannot write about it or recommend it after all. So while we have both found some great treatments and therapists this way, we have also had some *wojus* experiences.

As we were writing this section, we had to laugh at the amount of facials we've had over the years that have been simply shocking. We must have blocked them out in some kind of post-traumatic coping mechanism. We've been insulted by therapists about our skin, left salons after a 'deep cleanse' facial with our morning make-up still on and been stuck with lumps of exfoliator glued to the moisturiser slapped on by a decidedly uninterested beautician.

Aisling has suffered three black eyes after treatments: the first after slipping in a decidedly unsafe Cleopatra bath, the second after landing smack on the floor after the towel on the treatment bed slipped, and the third after falling while getting out of a floatation tank filled with slimy seaweed goo that had no rails to hang on to. She has even had lymphatic drainage that left her with bruises and has a grand dose of broken veins around her nose after a therapist scalded the life out of her skin with what felt like boiling water.

And fag fingers? We cannot count the times a therapist's fag smelling fingers and breath ruined the whole experience.

Now, who says we do not suffer for beauty?

But not to worry – this is an easily remedied problem. You can book in for a salon facial with someone who has been recommended, or you can simply replicate the steps they use at home, using your own products. A week or so of using a decent exfoliator, a face mask or two and a few early nights will soon sort you out.

Salon facials vary quite a bit depending on the ritual, technique or products used. On the most basic level they boil down to a thorough cleanse, followed by exfoliation, a mask or perhaps two, a facial massage and then all the usual stuff you'd do yourself anyway.

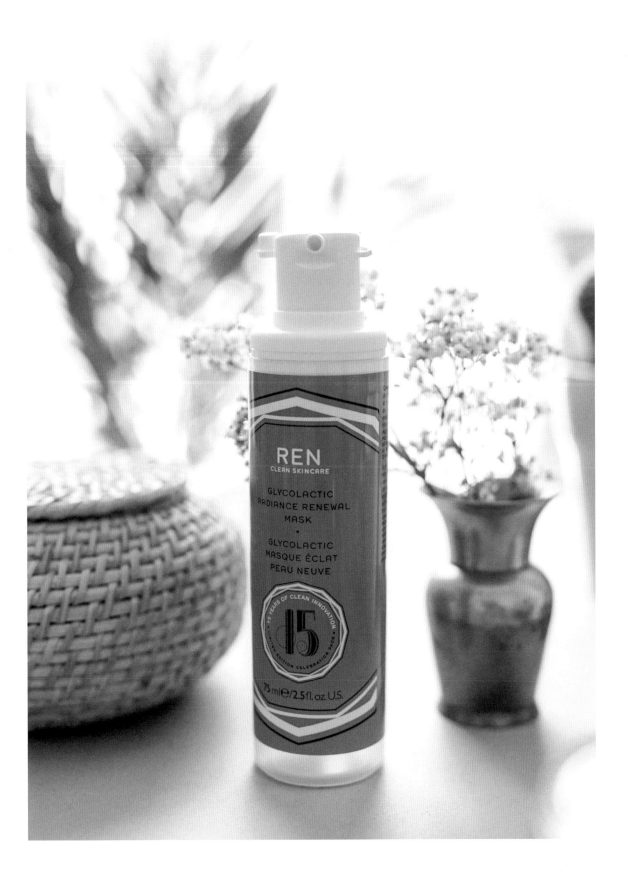

The mask is really the thing. Try a mask after your exfoliation – it works so much better when the product can actually sink into fresh skin. Choose your mask according to your skin concern.

PORE-CLEARING MASKS

Congested skin with blocked pores needs the tough stuff to suck all that gunk out of pores. You honestly can't beat a good old-fashioned mud mask and anything with kaolin or activated charcoal will unblock pores and soak up grease.

Origins Clear Improvement Activate Charcoal Mask will clear the pores and so will a cheap and cheerful sachet of Montague Jeunesse. Glamglow Youthmud Tinglexfoliate Treatment, which is the biggest example of hype and targeted marketing we've seen, is also fairly good at decongesting and clearing skin – but beware that you get very little for your money, as all their budget seems to have been spent on sending free samples to every blogger and Z-list celebrity in this galaxy and a few other galaxies not yet discovered. The tingle is down to the addition of glycolic acid in the mud, which you can get naturally from Irish brand Ógra and their Peat Face and Body Mask. If you want to use a glycolic mask, Ren Glycolactic Radiance Renewal Mask gets straight down to the task at hand: to give you better skin instantly. This mask gets your skin glowing with lots of exfoliating and brightening ingredients. It really is a hero product.

One of the very best skin-clearing masks is SkinCeuticals Clarifying Clay Masque, which deeply cleanses within pores with a 5% hydroxy acid blend.

No7 Beautiful Skin Vacuum Pore Mask, a gel-clay hybrid, peels off, unclogging pores as it goes, and will fill you with a delighted horror similar to the kind experienced when using a Bioré Deep Cleansing Pore Strip for the first time. All that disgusting gunk available for inspection? We're sold.

Ren Clarimatte Invisible Pores Detox Mask is another detoxifying clay mask that leaves pores appearing smaller and skin smoother. A great pore-clearer is Payot Detoxifying Radiance Mask, which Aisling uses way more often than she should, because she loves it so very much.

Alternatively, you can use masks with active enzymes, fruit acids or glycolics to clear skin. Elemis Fruit Active Rejuvenating Mask and Caudalie Instant Detox Mask are both great at nibbling away horrid grey skin.

MOISTURE MASKS

Great moisture masks abound if you are dry and dehydrated, and you can even use one right after your decongesting one to really make sure the lovely ingredients soak right in. Try a gel mask as they make great soothing and refreshing pick-me-ups – Charlotte Tilbury Multi-Miracle Glow Cleanser Mask & Balm and The Body Shop Drops of Youth Bouncy Sleeping Mask are both gorgeous big tubs of gloop that will instantly plump up skin. The Bio-essence Hydra Tri-Action Aqua Droplet Sleeping Beauty Mask (from Korea, of course) is something special: it contains two types of hyaluronic acid and when patted gently onto skin it instantly draws in water from the atmosphere, forming fat droplets on your face which you then massage in. It's addictive.

Some other sumptuous masks include Decléor Hydra Floral Multi-Protection Ultra-Moisturising & Plumping Expert Mask, Clinique Even Better Brightening Moisture Mask and Lancôme Hydra Intense Moisturising Gel Mask.

Overnight masks are the business, and while they've always been available, sleeping masks are definitely one of the next big things and we're going to see more and more of them.

Overnight masks are the business, and while they've always been available, sleeping masks are definitely one of the next big things and we're going to see more and more of them. Nars Aqua Gel Luminous Mask, Origins Drink Up Intensive, Clinique Moisture Surge Overnight Mask and Kiehl's Ultra Facial Overnight Hydrating Masque will transform your skin and banish fine lines.

Even the evil Period Face (page 89) can be tamed into submission with a mask, if you can drag yourself away from that half-kilo bar of Dairy Milk to slap one on your face. Instant brightening and smoothing is available via the miracles that are Dermalogica Multivitamin Power Recovery Masque and Origins GinZing Refreshing Face Mask.

When you've got rosacea-prone skin, sometimes only a good mask can soothe and calm the whole red mess right down. In times of crisis turn to Dr Andrew Weil for Origins Mega-Mushroom Skin Relief Face Mask or Avène Antirougeurs Calm Soothing Repair Mask. They will both work hard to tone down redness and relieve irritation and discomfort.

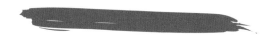

CHAPTER 4

· SERUM ·

We love serums. We love serums with the strength of a thousand suns and almost as much as Karl Lagerfeld loves Choupette and Donald Trump loves hairspray. Which is a whole lot.

For anyone who is not yet a convert, adding a serum to your routine means that you benefit from concentrated ingredients that work right on the surface of the skin to treat just about any skin concern that you have. The problem with serums is that there is no standardised definition of what they actually are and of what makes a product a serum as opposed to a runny moisturiser or a gloopy gel with loads of filler ingredients and very little of the good stuff.

It's almost as bad as flippin' Alphabet Creams (page 143). But creating consumer confusion is something that the cosmetic industry has refined to a fine art, so it is up to us to educate ourselves, read labels and figure out what is actually in this new 'wonder' product.

The easiest thing to do is to glance down the ingredient list (which will be printed in the smallest type ever, so you'll have to get out your magnifying glass) and see where in the list the 'actives' are.

The active ingredients are the ones that actually do something, instead of the ones that are just there to keep the mixture stable or to make it easy to apply, such as silicones. So, for example, if a serum advertises itself as a moisturising hyaluronic acid serum, but you can clearly see that hyaluronic acid is sixth on the list of eight ingredients, then the amount of hyaluronic acid it contains is minimal and you're being deliberately deceived. It doesn't matter what the active is – it could be lactic or glycolic acid, vitamin C or any expensive ingredient – reading the label will tell you exactly how much of it is in there.

Put serum on after your cleanser (and toner, if you use it). Let it sink in for a couple of minutes and then apply moisturiser.

So now all that is out of the way, let's see which serums are actually great for your skin.

The best serums

You can use any serum at any age – they treat skin concerns rather than rigid age groups. It doesn't matter if something markets itself 'for the quarter-life crisis' or any of that lark – if you like the look of the ingredients and think it will do your skin good, then go for it. It's easy to spend a fortune on serum because if it's good, it will have a high concentration of quality actives. The cheaper serums tend to rely more on inexpensive ingredients, like glycerin and silicones, which actually are very good at moisturising and should not be written off, particularly if you have normal skin.

ALL-ROUNDERS

Brands like Nivea have great serums – their Cellular Anti-Age Skin-Refining Serum is fresh, light and will make your skin feel better straight away. Use it under the night moisturiser from the same range and you have a duo that is perfect for hydration on a budget. Don't turn your nose up at the supermarket brands either: check the ingredients and if they have hyaluronic acid, niacin or glycerin, they are going to hydrate and smooth your skin.

Olay are leaders in the mid-market skincare field and some of their serums are fantastic. There are so many of them, so choose one from the Total Effects line. Give the moisturising and serum duo a bash – it's great for busy mornings when you don't have time to layer up your products. No7 Protect & Perfect Advanced cannot go without a mention either: they've done the research and presented us with the evidence that their serums really do work. Boots Botanics Radiant Youth Super Serum is another serum we can really get on board with – it is absolutely excellent for the price point.

Oskia Super 16 Pro-Collagen Super Serum will work happily with any skin regime as it contains a gentle retinol ingredient and other nutrients. Laura Mercier Multi-Vitamin Serum is a duo crammed with antioxidant vitamins A, C and E, which protect skin against damage. And other all-rounders like Origins Plantscription Youth-renewing Face Oil, Aesop Parsley Seed Anti-Oxidant Serum, Clinique Smart Custom-Repair Serum and Omorovicza Radiance Renewal Serum all work well to give dull skin its mojo back.

Although Bobbi Brown are better known for their make-up, some of their skincare is very good. The Intensive Skin Supplement is a great serum. BareMinerals Active Cell Renewal Night Serum is another good skincare product from a make-up brand.

Don't turn your nose up at the supermarket brands: check the ingredients and if they have hyaluronic acid, niacin or glycerin, they are going to hydrate and smooth your skin.

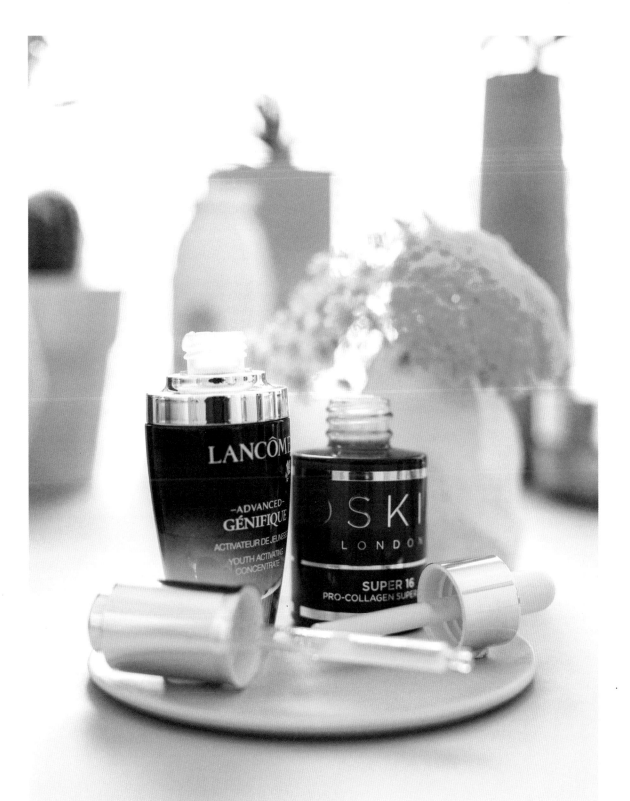

OILY SKIN

Oily, acne-prone skin is well catered for on the serum front as not only can serums produce a potent mix of skin-friendly ingredients, they often also contain glycolic and salicylic acid, which work quietly away all day and night on your skin without harshness. Clinique Turnaround Revitalizing Serum with salicylic acid and Estée Lauder Perfectionist [CP+R] Wrinkle-Lifting/Firming Serum are both stand-outs. Thalgo Intense Regulating Serum works very hard to calm down bad-tempered skin as does Murad T-Zone Pore Refining Serum.

DRY SKIN

Those with dry skin should head straight towards serums packed with hyaluronic acid and other water attracters. When you put your moisturiser on top of the serum, it seals in the serum's hydration, leaving your skin feeling soft and nourished for the day or night. Fine lines will magically disappear, your skin will look softer and fresher and make-up will go on much more smoothly. No one is paying us to say this: it really happens. These serums work well after a period of illness too and will go a long way towards restoring your skin to normal.

Serums do exist that consist solely of hyaluronic acid but through trial and error, we've found that hyaluronic acid feels more moisturising and performs more effectively when it is mixed with other ingredients. If you are hell-bent on using pure hyaluronic acid, it looks and feel exactly like water. To use it, you dampen your face and pat it on. It is not until you apply moisturiser over the top that you

Fine lines will magically disappear, your skin will look softer and fresher and make-up will go on much more smoothly. No one is paying us to say this: it really happens.

will notice any benefits – the hyaluronic acid needs to draw in moisture to work.

However, as we've said we prefer hyaluronic acid serums that contain other complementary ingredients such as vitamin E or resveratrol. Hydrating serums we like (and boy, was it hard to whittle down this list) include Oz Naturals Hyaluronic Acid + Vitamin C Professional Moisturizing Serum, SkinCeuticals Hydrating B5 Gel, Olay Regenerist 3 Point Super Serum, Shiseido Bio-Performance Glow Revival Serum, Clarins Double Serum, The Body Shop Vitamin E Overnight Serum-in-Oil and Trilogy Nutrient Plus Firming Serum. They all give skin that's gasping like a landed fish some aqua back.

Alpha H is one of the serum brands that are creating the most excitement at the moment, but its original formula is strong so it can only be used on alternate nights due to its high concentration of glycolic acid. Liquid Gold Intensive Night Repair Serum, on the other hand, can be used nightly, and we think it is a better alternative. For a gentler approach – but one we think is underrated for its efficacy – try Ren Radiance Perfection Serum.

MATURE SKIN

We're saying post-thirty-five as a rough guideline, but you can use the following serums at any age. It's important to remember that you can use any product at any age, so don't let labels and marketing upset you or make you feel boxed into a type or make you think you need more even if everything is working fine. The purpose of good skincare should be to make you feel great about yourself and if you feel miserable about using a product labelled 'mature', then simply don't do it.

If you turn your back on products labelled 'mature' or 'anti-ageing' though, you might be missing out because with these serums, we're really sucking diesel as they tend to have a higher amount of active ingredients. 'Mature' and 'anti-ageing' serums are among the most brilliant products around and can seriously supercharge your skincare routine. You're quite literally spoilt

When you put your moisturiser on top of the serum, it seals in the serum's hydration, leaving your skin feeling soft and nourished for the day or night.

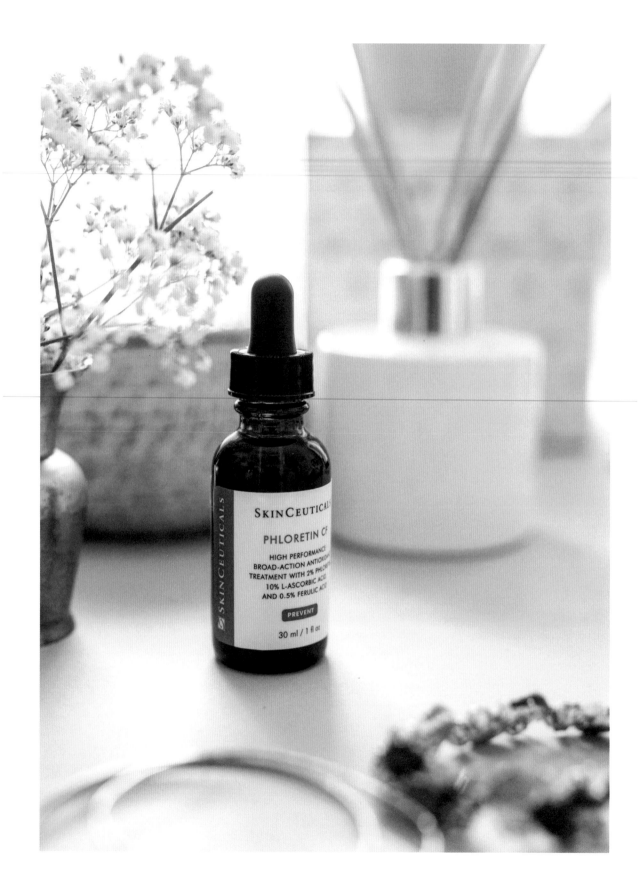

If you turn your back on products labelled 'mature' or 'pro-ageing', you might be missing out because with these serums, we're really sucking diesel as they tend to have a higher amount of active ingredients.

for choice, but be warned: the cosmetic industry views you as the segment of the market that is ready to spend on premium products, so make sure you don't fall for marketing hype.

Estée Lauder Advanced Night Repair is one of the originals and it is still one of the best, while Pevonia Power Repair Age Correction Collagen & Myoxy Caviar Intensifier is an absolute treat for skin. It is so deeply hydrating, and this nutrient-rich serum really does saturate skin with moisture. We almost wept when it was finished. Another serum that will cause you to weep when it is gone is SkinCeuticals Resveratrol B E, which Aisling loved so much she almost *scweamed* and *scweamed* when it was empty. L'Oréal Youth Code Serum, L'Oréal Age Perfect Intensive Re-Nourish Serum and Olay 3 Point Super Serum have all also been used to the very last drops.

CHAPTER 5

· MOISTURISER ·

Moisturiser has changed and upped its game. Due to healthy competition from serums that contain so many concentrated actives, a lot of people began to wonder if they even needed to bother with a decent moisturiser any more. After all, they were getting everything they needed from their serums and oils, right? Well, not exactly. Moisturiser might not sit right on top of the skin any more but that doesn't mean it doesn't have a lot to offer beside being a mere emollient.

The cosmetic industry has been busy and has set to work to create a whole different class of moisturiser with lots of extra skincare benefits. Active ingredients such as retinol, antioxidants and tons of niacin, silicones and other ingredients improve the look, feel and pleasure of using the product. Now moisturisers brighten the look of skin, blur lines and imperfections and, with the emergence of CC and BB hybrids, double up as light foundations too. Moisturiser is carving out a new niche for itself and it will continue to improve.

Beauty decoded: Topical

'Topical' just means applied to the surface of the skin – so moisturiser is a topical product. Botox, on the other hand, is an injectable, and injectable products are the only ones that can penetrate the surface of the skin. The only ones. Think about it. The skin is a tremendously successful organ and it has many functions. But one of its primary tasks is to keep our insides inside and potential toxins and harmful substances out. It does this by being remarkably difficult to penetrate and there is no skincare molecule which can penetrate the surface of the skin. (See page 55 for more on this.)

When discussing creams and serums, the cosmetics industry deliberately tries to confuse us by using such vague language that it may seem as though our chosen product can actually penetrate the skin and work wonders beneath the surface, but now you know it can't.

The best moisturisers

Using moisturiser and the benefits you feel it brings you depend very much upon your skin type. Drier and mature skin will often feel uncomfortable and unhappy without the application of a rich moisturiser immediately after cleansing. We know that the phrase 'quite literally' is overused, and often incorrectly. But in this case, we think we can confidently say that some people would *quite literally* lose their lives without their daily dose of creamy goodness. Yes, there would be *literal* cases of dead bodies piled on the streets with shrivelled-up faces. Drier skin types can get through bucket-loads of the stuff and even oily skin types are usually inextricably attached to their twice-daily dose of moisturiser.

DAY MOISTURISERS

Day moisturisers should have a couple of essential properties: a good SPF, a nice formula that will sit well on the skin and provide a good base for make-up and some antioxidants to provide an extra layer of protection against those 'external aggressors' (pollution and the weather) that are so bad for skin. Quite often, day moisturisers can be great multitaskers, doubling up as foundation primers and containing that all important line blurring effect. CC creams have further added to the blurred lines between skincare and colour cosmetics in a non-pervy Robin Thicke fashion by evening out skin tone while they're at it.

So, let's have a look at what's worth the spend.

NORMAL SKIN

L'Occitane Pivoine Sublime Perfecting Essence works well for normal skin and Nude Skincare Radiant Day Moisturizer is a good brightening option for this skin type. Lancôme Bienfait Multi-Vital SPF Sunscreen is a solid sun-shielding moisturiser, while Lancôme Energie de Vie Dullness Relief & Energy Recharge Daily Lotion-in-Gel is a super-fresh take on moisturiser that instantly hydrates. Mac Mineralize Timecheck Lotion is light and refreshing and works well as a primer under make-up too. Avène Hydrance Optimale UV Light Hydrating Cream is a firm

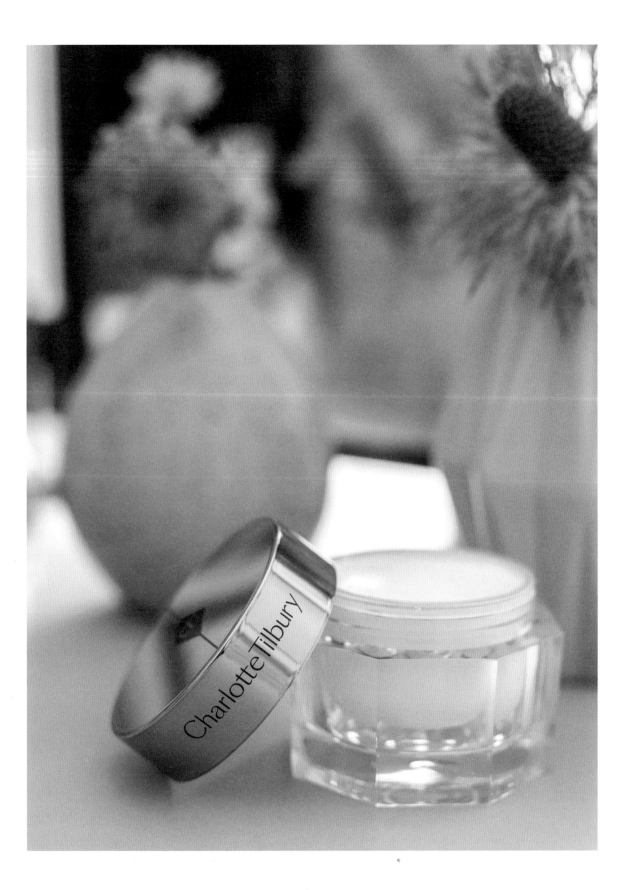

Bargain beauty: From moisturiser to hand lotion

Dermatologists say they can tell a woman's age immediately by looking at her hands, because we tend to look after our faces much more than our paws. Throw them off the scent by always using SPF on your *lámhs* as well as your face, neck and chest. If you buy a face product that you don't like or that stings the eyes off you, make sure that serum or moisturiser doesn't go to waste. Rub it into hands, nails, elbows and hooves. It's much better than dumping it.

And if you are buying a special hand product, Aveda Hand Relief Moisturizing Creme and Burt's Bees Almond Milk Beeswax Hand Creme are fantastic.

favourite with normal skin types at the less expensive segment of the market. And you know what? The Aldi Lacura moisturisers are constantly rated as a good choice by many women and having used them, we agree. Nivea, Boots, Essentials and supermarket own brands all have decent choices too.

OILY SKIN

Good day moisturisers for oily and combination skin include Clinique Even Better Skin Tone Correcting Lotion and Estée Lauder DayWear Advanced Multi-Protection Anti-Oxidant Creme. Murad Oil-Control Mattifier is great for dampening down shine and with lots of beneficial ingredients including willow bark, which helps to clear skin of impurities and reduces the possibility of breakouts. There are some great budget-friendly options for oily skin types in the Bioderma and Garnier ranges, so make sure to check these out. Just remember the golden rule – avoid alcohol-heavy formulas.

DRY SKIN

Dry and mature skin can give it a little more kick with moisturising choices. Clinique's Moisture Surge Extended Thirst Relief, Clarins Gentle Day Cream for Sensitive Skin, Prevage Anti-Aging Moisture Cream Broad Spectrum Sunscreen and Laura Mercier Tinted Moisturizer are all worth checking out. Kiehl's Powerful Wrinkle Reducing Cream is a joy to use if you have dry skin, as is Marks & Spencer Formula Advanced Cosmetox+ Wrinkle Decrease Night Cream and Nivea Cellular Anti-Age Skin-Refining Serum. Clinique Dramatically Different Moisturizing Lotion helps strengthen skin's own moisture barrier by over 50% so more moisture stays locked in, which is great if you are using it over moisture-rich serum and oil.

MATURE SKIN

You won't go far wrong with the Olay Total Effects range, particularly the Total Effects 7-in-1 Anti-Ageing Moisturiser. Dermalogica Pure Light is pricey, but it does have an SPF 50 and is light and easily absorbed so that make-up sits well on top of it. Olay Regenerist Luminous Brightening & Protecting Lotion with Sunscreen is a solid choice, as are the moisturisers from the No7 Perfect & Protect Advanced line.

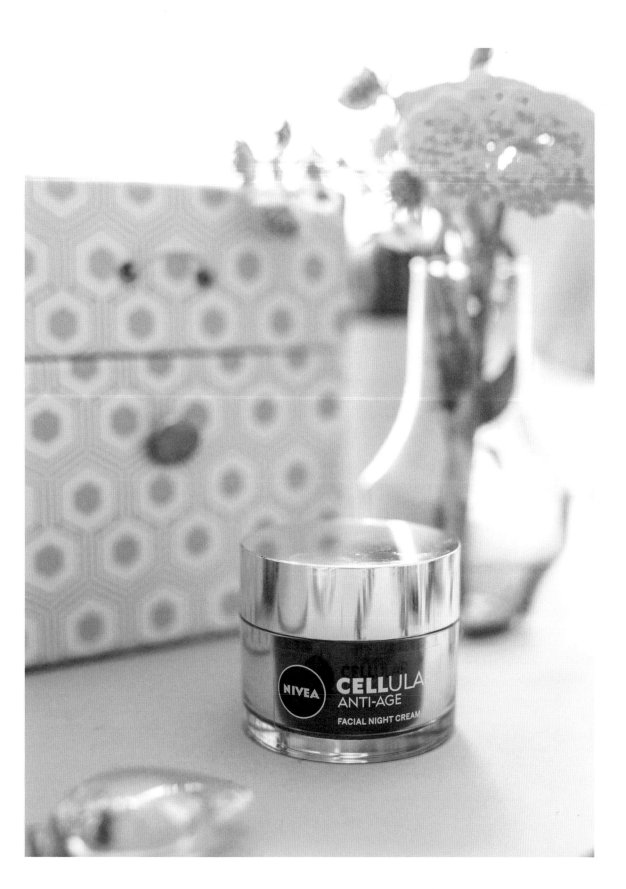

Remember – if it has SPF and antioxidant vitamins (particularly vitamin C, the skin brightener) you can't really go wrong, no matter what the price point it. That budget moisturiser you pick up in the supermarket will be just as good for layering and sealing in your other skincare, as long as it suits your skin. Vitamin C offers sun protection as well, so it's a great ingredient to have in a day moisturiser.

NIGHT MOISTURISERS

With night moisturisers, it's often a case of the richer the better, but you have a couple of options. If your skin is young, oily or normal, you might want to skip the night moisturiser (and oil) altogether and just go with serum. It's completely up to you – if your skin feels overloaded, then don't use a night moisturiser.

Many night creams are too rich and heavy for younger or oily skin anyway. Try a light night cream instead, like No7 Early Defence Night Cream: the light, almost gel-like texture of this cream makes it a refreshing night-time solution. The Body Shop Vitamin C Glow Boosting Moisturiser is another good option.

If on the other hand your skin is dry, dehydrated or mature, we can definitely say that investing in a good night moisturiser is one of the best things you can do for your skin. It will seal in all the magic of your serum. If you find the consistency of the cream too thick, just use a tiny bit and mix it with your facial oil.

Ren Frankincense Revitalising Night Cream, Lancôme Genifique Repair Youth Activating Night Cream, Elemis Pro-Collagen Marine Cream and Indeed Labs Fillume Volumising Moisturiser are all great night moisturisers, and Eucerin Even Brighter Night Cream even helps to clear up sun spots too.

Decléor Hydra Floral Multi-Protection 24hr Moisture Activator Light Cream and Nip+Fab Viper Venom Extreme Night Fix Skin-Perfecting Night Cream hydrate your skin as you snooze, while Bioderma Atoderm Intensive Soothing Emollient Care will help with extremely dry, flaky or patchy skin – just make sure you exfoliate or tone first to give the moisturiser a chance to sink into your skin.

If we won the Euromillions, it would be Giorgio Armani Crema Nera all the way – there was almost a breakdown of epic proportions in one writer's house the night it ran out. It's superb, rich and oh so dense. If you love richer than rich night creams, you'll also love Lancôme Rénergie Nuit Multi-Lift Lifting Firming Anti-Wrinkle Night Cream. Darphin also have some great rich moisturisers, including Fibrogene Line Response Nourishing Cream. Aveda Botanical Kinetics Intense Hydrating Rich Creme is another brilliant night moisturiser that works for us on the thick and luxurious front. Oily and acne-prone skin will get on well with Clinique Super Rescue Antioxidant Night Moisturizer.

Night time is the best time for retinol-based products. Applying them during the day makes skin too sensitive to the sun so stick to antioxidants for the day and retinol for night. This Works Extreme Night Cream, SkinCeuticals Retinol 0.3, Indeed Labs Retinol Reface Skin Resurfacer and Roc Deep Wrinkle Night Cream all contain retinol, albeit in much lower concentrations than you'll get from a dermatologist, but there is evidence to show that even at these levels retinol can work (for more on the best pro-ageing ingredients, see page 56).

Beauty decoded: Peptides and collagen - does my molecule look big in this?

Peptides have long been championed by the cosmetics industry as the next coming of Skincare Christ and extraordinary pro-ageing promises are attached to their presence in lotions and potions. They're mini-proteins formed when collagen breaks down, and the theory is that adding them to skin creams can trick the skin into thinking it needs to produce more collagen, which makes it look younger, plumper and more hydrated.

Almost all molecules are just too big to squeeze through the skin's barrier and, by and large, peptides fall into this category. In theory, they can do all the things the label says they do – but 'in theory' is not the same as actually doing it on your face. They can't fill in lines and act like Botox or filler – nothing that's not injected can. Oh and collagen? Same story here as peptides, unfortunately. It doesn't matter how much collagen is crammed into your cream; it's just going to sit on the surface of your skin and not do much else. It simply can't penetrate the epidermis, so you'll need to get collagen injections to see any benefits.

But the new next-gen peptides are improving and becoming tinier, so we won't write them off just yet. If you really, really, really, really want to try a peptide-based formulation, go for products from Olay Regenerist, which contains matrixyl, or No7 Protect & Perfect,

both massively popular ranges. And although Indeed Labs Snoxin Facial Line Fighter sounds like something you might blow into a tissue during a nasty cold, it is actually a highly concentrated blast of peptides that swears on its mother's life it can improve every aspect of skin ageing from crows' feet to jowls.

Even though peptides can't actually penetrate the skin, there is now some evidence that they may help other ingredients work more effectively, so we won't rule them out completely for now.

But we're keeping a good eye on you, peptides. We still don't trust you.

Eye cream

Ah, eye creams. How you continue to survive in your astronomically priced, tiny jars never ceases to amaze us. You are a true triumph of myth, marketing and habit superseding all forms of common sense and actual benefits.

It is certainly true that the skin under the eyes is super-thin and very sensitive and does need a degree of attention that differs from the rest of your face. We're not arguing with that. As it lacks oil, it does need to be helped along to stay well-nourished and well-balanced – but you don't necessarily need a specialised product to do that.

No one actually needs to use eye cream, but it's not advisable either to bring heavy moisturisers right under your eyes as they can drag down the skin, possibly cause milia (little white lumps) and irritate your eyes. Instead, try using your regular oil or serum, bringing it right up to your socket and patting some of it under your eyes. Even if an oil or serum says 'avoid the eye area', it is usually okay to use it under the eyes unless it is actually made out of Domestos or similar.

Burning, stinging eyes are no joke, so avoid products with fragrance if you have sensitivity issues, and only use a moisturiser you already know suits your skin. A good trick to avoid irritation is to use creams only around your orbital area (you can feel it with your fingers – it's the bone running around your eyes) and let the cream 'creep' up by itself. Forget all the talk about 'cross hatching' and 'lymphatic drainage' application methods, which just makes things needlessly complicated.

Of course many people want to use an eye cream anyway. In that case, we suggest you try a serum eye product instead as they are lighter and reduce the risk of overloading the skin under your eyes (plus we just love serums).

Good ingredients to look out for are hyaluronic acid to instantly hydrate, caffeine to help firm and depuff, and antioxidants (vitamins A, C and E), which can help prevent further damage. Trilogy Age Proof CoQ10 Eye Recovery Concentrate, Estée Lauder Advanced Night Repair Eye Serum and Kiehl's Super Multi-Corrective Eye-Opening Serum are all great.

And if you want to splash out, the sky is the limit with eye serums. One of the best fancypants ones, which works particularly well for mature skin, is Lancôme Absolue Yeux Precious Cells Global Multi-Restorative Eye Concentrate. If you have just won the Euromillions, Bioeffect EGF Cellular Activating Serum is the absolute stand-out eye serum.

Alas, there's no product that can get rid of dark circles, because they are either genetic or the result of too little sleep or an underlying health concern. Obviously, they will not respond to any amount of over-the-counter topical preparations. However, eye products with built-in concealer are very useful for dealing with them. If an eye product promises 'instant radiance' or 'instant dark circle reduction', that means that the product contains concealer. For a great concealing eye cream, try Estée Lauder Idealist Cooling Eye Illuminator, Kiehl's Clearly Corrective Dark Circle Perfector, Garnier BB Cream Miracle Skin Perfector Eye Roll-On, No7 Youthful Eye Serum or Olay Regenerist Luminous Dark Circle Correcting Swirl.

Beauty decoded: Best pro-ageing ingredients

If you want to use products that will really work and cut through all the marketing bull, then these are the ingredients. No made-up science here – these guys have been proven to give results.

AHAS

Alpha hydroxy acids, such as glycolic acid and lactic acid, work by dissolving dead skin cells and lifting them off the skin. These chemical exfoliants are always preferable to scratchy scrubs as they're kinder to skin (see page 20 for more). They may also stimulate collagen production (studies of this are currently underway) but they do reduce the appearance of fine lines and make the skin stronger. Using a good AHA will make your skin look instantly fresher and younger. Research on this has been ongoing in our bathroom cabinets for some time.

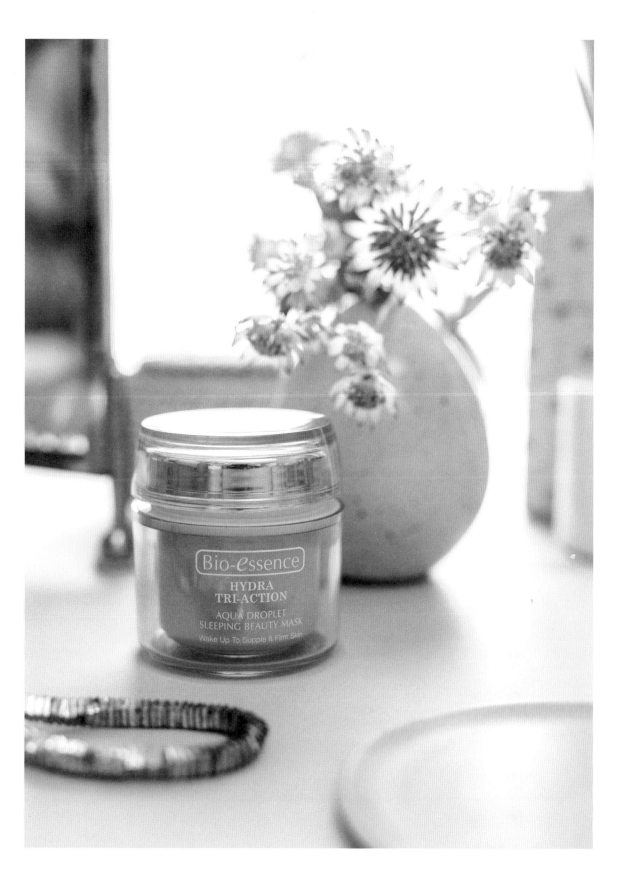

ANTIOXIDANTS

We all know we need a good helping of antioxidants in our diet to stay healthy (so eat up those Brussel sprouts, you hear) and they work wonders on the skin too. Vitamin A is key to retinol, vitamin B3 to niacin, and the antioxidant vitamins C and E are pretty powerful too. Add co-enzyme Q-10 and ferulic acid to the mix and you've got yourself some of the best ingredients to keep skin performing well.

BOTOX

No matter how many creams and serums exist with sciencey-sounding Botoxy names, they are not Botox and we wish they would just shut up and go away. Thousands of people are fooled by 'Botox in a jar' claims and as they often cost the equivalent of the GDP of a small country, they are a complete rip-off. There will never be Botox in a jar because it is an injectable ingredient that should only be administered by a trained practitioner. The fact that real Botox is often overused, or used by beauticians who are not properly trained and don't have a breeze what they are doing, is not the fault of Botox. It is up to you to check out the credentials of your practitioner (who should ideally be a dermatologist).

Botox works. We're all for choosing whichever treatment you find works best, and if you'd like to try Botox or already use it and find it works for you then go for it.

You will not end up looking like Joan Rivers (RIP), because she had a ton of plastic surgery, or be unable to move your face if you get a subtle course of injections to soften lines.

HYALURONIC ACID

The best ingredient to pull moisture from the air and into your skin. Instant results. Instant happiness. It's the best thing to happen since sliced bread and the best thing to happen to skincare since ... ever.

NIACIN

A form of vitamin B3, niacin is an increasingly popular skincare ingredient. Until relatively recently, the molecules in niacin were considered too large to be absorbed through the skin –

Thousands of people are fooled by 'Botox in a jar' claims and as they often cost the equivalent of the GDP of a small country, they are a complete rip-off.

and they still are, no matter what you'll read to the contrary. But now you'll see this ingredient used in loads of dry skin and pro-ageing products because it works really well to lock in moisture, reduce hyperpigmentation and soothe irritated skin. It's also great for rosacea and acne.

RETINOL

Another vitamin-derived ingredient, this time a form of vitamin A, retinol is probably the best ingredient for mature skin as it can actually reverse the signs of ageing, resurface the skin, boost collagen production and blast age spots into oblivion.

But of course there is a downside or else we'd be covered from head to toe in the stuff 24/7. It can irritate the hell out of your skin, which is why most topical preparations only contain miniscule amounts, so sensitive types should approach with extreme caution. Look out for retinyl palmitate and retinylaldehyde in ingredient lists – they're a milder form of the full strength version and take longer to work but they're good for at-home use. We find that it is best to use products containing retinol or its derivatives at night, as retinol makes your skin sensitive to sun damage, and make sure to use lots of high strength SPF during the day.

A full strength dose of retinol can only be prescribed by a dermatologist, so if you want to go hard you'll have to make an appointment. Or go home.

SPF

Sorry to harp on about this, but here it comes again anyway. It actually doesn't matter how many fancypants serums and creams you plaster all over your face if you're not using sunscreen. We can thank the sun for 80% of the visible signs of ageing – think about that and don't skip the sunscreen.

Retinol is probably the best ingredient for mature skin as it can actually reverse the signs of ageing, resurface the skin, boost collagen production and blast age spots into oblivion.

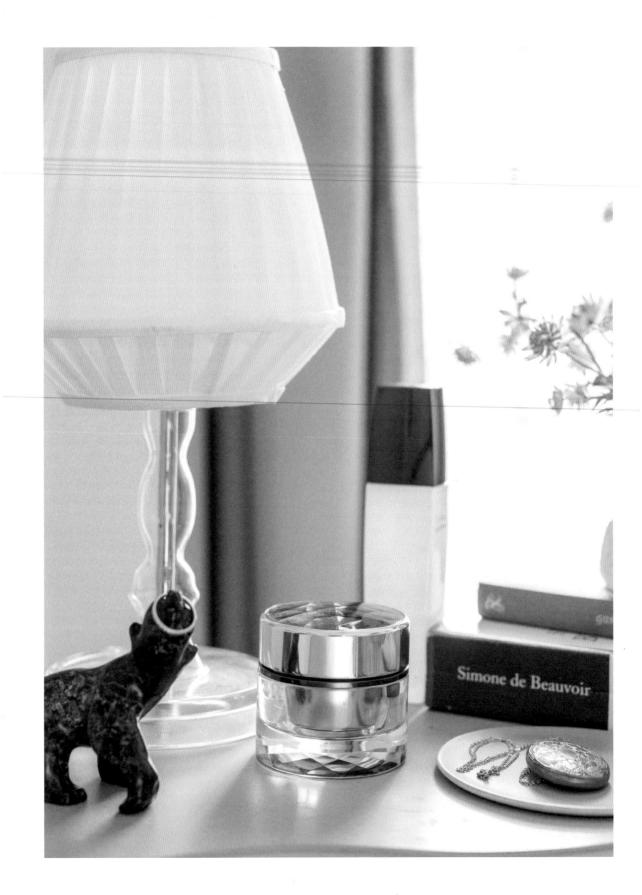

Beauty decoded: Pillow Face

Beware of Hollywood stars who swear on their lives that they've tried Botox once, didn't like it and so never got it done again. We are somehow supposed to believe that ageing hasn't changed them and they just naturally look thirty-five. Jennifer Aniston is probably the best example of these downright lies: she went from looking disturbingly similar to Iggy Pop to a chubby-cheeked twenty-something overnight.

Pillow Face occurs when plumping ingredients are injected into the face to counteract loss of fullness. It makes the Pillow-Faced person look remarkably smooth of face – and when overdone, it looks plain ridiculous, more like a round cushion with two small buttons for eyes than a pillow really. Everyone in Hollywood over forty who manages to stay a size zero while maintaining the cherubic face of a two-year-old is probably a fan of injectables.

You don't have to go for such a drastic change but a course of hyaluronic acid injections or other face plumpers can instantly refresh and plump up skin.

~~~

Beware of Hollywood stars who swear on their lives that they've tried Botox once, didn't like it and so never got it done again.

~~~

CHAPTER 6

· FACIAL OIL ·

Facial oils are the absolute shiz. Leave your assumptions about putting oil on your face right at the door. That's it. Actually put those assumptions outside the door and *dún* that *doras*. If you want instant skincare gratification, you'll get it with an oil. Your skin will immediately become more supple and smooth without any fancy science or crazy claims. Fact.

There is really no doubt about it: facial oils are brilliant. They are loaded with naturally occurring fatty acids, antioxidants like vitamins A, C and E and often have antibacterial properties. As a result of this, they are a powerhouse in the moisturising, nourishing and softening stakes and are generally really, really nice to skin.

The best facial oils

Most oils are blends so there are some that are great all-rounders and others that suit some skin types better than others. Dry skin benefits from almost all and any oil in existence, but sensitive and oily types can also have their day in court as there are lots of oils out there for you too.

Many people find night-time use of oils sufficient and unless you have dry skin, it's probably fine to skip day-time use. At night, use a couple of drops of facial oil either mixed with your moisturiser or patted lightly on top of it for extra hydration. If you're applying oil in the morning, make sure to mix it with you moisturiser as foundation does not sit well on a bed of oil.

BEST FOR NORMAL SKIN

If you have normal skin, it is already perfectly balanced and you probably don't need an oil at all. But if you would like to use one, go for it – it can only do your skin good. Mix a drop or two in with your moisturiser at night for extra hydration. Choose any light oil – Ren, Origins, L'Oréal and Lancôme all do nice non-greasy oils. You can take your pick – just don't overdo it.

BEST FOR OILY SKIN

Although it seems counterintuitive, do not write off facial oils if your skin is oily as they can calm it down and stop it from panicking and over-producing sebum. Using oil can actually stop the production of more oil – use a scant drop of oil and you won't overload your skin.

It was Dr Hauschka who famously said 'treat like with like', and we bow to the great Doc on this (even though we don't agree at all with some of his other 'rules'). Oily skin is fond of acting like a stroppy teen, no matter what your age, and flies into a greasy rage when you dry it out. Use a light oil blend to reassure it that all is fine and there's no need to go into overdrive.

The right type of oil is important as heavy blends may sink into pores and clog up them up. Dr Hauschka Normalizing Day Oil is ideal, as are Boots Botanics Organic Facial Oil, Caudalie Overnight Vinosource Recover Oil and Darphin Niaouli Aromatic Care. Decléor Aromessence Ylang Ylang Purifying Serum gets on well with most oily skin, but be careful if you have sensitive skin as its loaded with aromatics.

Most women love rosehip oils with good reason – they're great for all skin types, moisturise well due to a high concentration of essential fatty acids, have antibacterial properties and can help to clear up scars, spots and blemishes. Pai, Trilogy and Kinvara (which is a great oil/serum hybrid) all make excellent rosehip oils.

Beauty tip: Oil and make-up

Oil makes a terrible base for make-up. Don't put make-up on directly over oil or it will cause everything to slide and creep and look shiny. You need to put a barrier of moisturiser over oil to seal it in and then you're away on a hack.

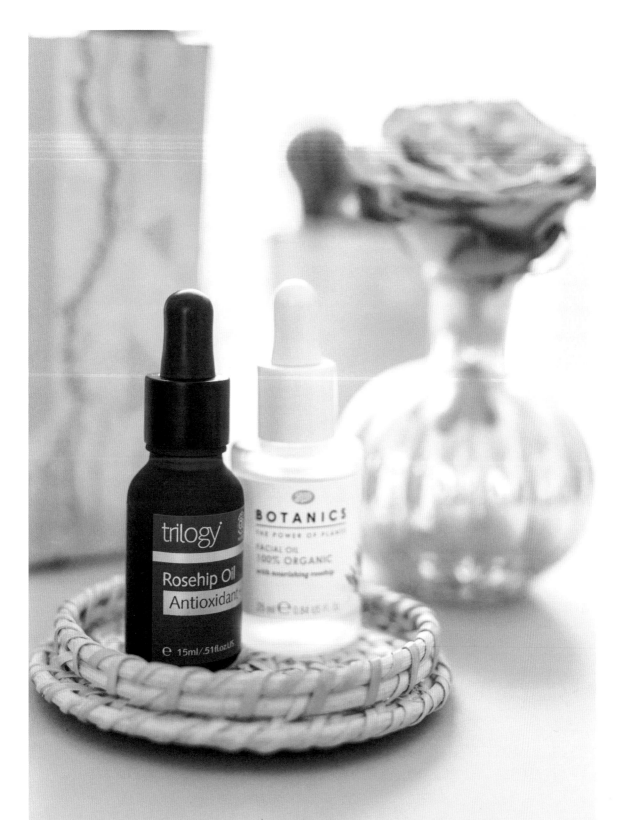

BEST FOR DRY SKIN

Dry skin lacks oil and literally sucks up the additional pure moisture from facial oils. We can't beg dry skin types enough to add one to your routine. A rich oil, used twice daily, will provide instant results that will continue to improve the suppleness and elasticity of your skin over time. Argan oil, in particular, is a very good moisturising ingredient as it has a high concentration of fatty acids and vitamin E, which makes it perfect for age support.

There is no shortage of luxury oils that have stood the test of time for a reason: Clarins Blue Orchid Face Treatment Oil and Kiehl's Midnight Recovery Concentrate are classics. Nude ProGenius Omega Treatment Oil, Sisley Black Rose Precious Face Oil and Sunday Riley Juno Hydroactive Cellular Face Oil are all expensive, but oh so worth it.

While Aisling's very dry skin drinks up oil quicker than a cat hoovers up a tin of tuna, she does have her special favourite. She loves rich oils and Darphin do the best – their Essential Oil Elixirs are fantastic with a blend for every skin type and their 8-Flower Nectar is amazing. Yes, you might have to sell off one of your children or start eating beans on toast to afford it but your skin will love you.

Oskia Restoration Oil is one of our favourites for night-time use, and Rodial Stemcell Super-Food Facial Oil and Clinique Turnaround Revitalizing Treatment Oil are day-time faves as they are lighter and better for use under make-up. Sunday Riley oils are amazing – just don't be put off by the smell, which it must be said is dreadful. We are not the only ones to think they smell like poo. Who says we don't have to suffer for beauty, eh? Some of the best mid-price oils we have used are Nourish Argan Skin Rescue Treatment and Úna Brennan Super Facialist Vitamin C+ Brighten Skin Renew Cleansing Oil, but there is an even cheaper alternative you might like.

Bargain beauty: Kitchen oils

Open your kitchen cupboard. Olive and coconut oils are rich natural moisturisers, but be warned – they are only really suitable for very dry skin.

BEST FOR SENSITIVE SKIN

Although it is more difficult to recommend an oil for sensitive types because body chemistry is so unique and what calms down the skin of one person may send another into a screaming rage, we'll give it our best shot. Rosehip oils are suitable for even the most sensitive skin, and rosacea often responds well too. Camomile blends are also soothing – Darphin Chamomile Aromatic Care will help to soothe and rebalance sensitive skin.

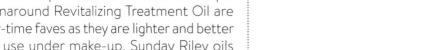

Beauty tip: Use oil to calm down spots

Laura was a lucky teenager. Although she suffered from horrendous fashion choices, was permanently embarrassed about the fact of her very existence and had ridiculous hair, she did possess one enviable thing that most of the rest of us didn't. While we were bawling in front of the mirror over the size of our spots, she had the most precious thing of all for a teenager: great skin.

So imagine her horror when, aged twenty, just as she was working out the general awkwardness and terrible hair situation (orange is a bad colour for her by the way), she was diagnosed with adult acne. What a kick in the fanny.

Cue several years of extreme self-consciousness and disgruntlement at the injustice of it all. And while trying to sort the problem out with doctors and medication, she resigned herself to covering it as well as she could with make-up and trying not to feel too desperate about herself.

We all know how hard it is not to direct all conversation towards that fascinating, glowing red bump on someone's chin, even when we try not to. Actually, especially when we try not to. We imagine it must be like a man trying not to have a sneaky look at a woman's cleavage and being caught in the act.

So we understand the agony of adult acne only too well and the importance of subduing that red angry face. Our number one tip has to be: make the spots easier to conceal.

If you use topical treatments laced with alcohol, they will dry out the surface skin of a blemish and make it much harder to cover. A sore, flaky (but still bulbous and red) blemish will drive you even crazier than the original spot did. So if you're using an alcohol-heavy prescription treatment, be sure to apply a facial oil of your choice on top. Good old-fashioned olive oil will do just fine too.

Alcohol robs your oily, blemish-prone skin of oil and ironically encourages your skin's oil production to go into overdrive (see page 21 for more). Smothering the blemish with oil counteracts any effects of alcohol and brings the pimple to a head in a pleasingly gross manner, making it safe to squeeze without making your skin even oilier. And now you can have all the fun of splatting it against the mirror. You can thank us later.

More importantly, once you've got smooth, unbroken skin on the surface of your breakout, you can cover it without much trouble. Check out the 'Concealer' section on page 148 to learn how.

If you're using an alcohol-heavy prescription treatment, be sure to apply a facial oil of your choice on top. Good old-fashioned olive oil will do just fine too.

CHAPTER 7

· SPF ·

SPF is key in protecting your skin from ageing. The sun is the biggest single cause of skin ageing. Forget genetics, forget smoking, forget everything else you've ever been told. While these things are very important, it's sun exposure that ages you quicker than anything else. Sitting in the sun is the skincare equivalent of putting salt on a slug. And if we can't appeal to your vanity, maybe we can appeal to your 1 in 50 chance of getting skin cancer.

The Irish Cancer Society is blue in the face telling us that we need to protect our skin from the sun. Irish people have the highest rate of skin cancer in Europe and it is the most common type of cancer in Ireland. The popularity of sun holidays has caused the skin cancer rate to soar – but even at home we need to be careful.

Dermatologists give different answers as to how much SPF you need to apply during the winter (October to March), ranging from none to SPF 15. You can normally pick up this level from your moisturiser or foundation. We get precious little sun during these months and in fact blocking the bit of it we do get may not be that beneficial. But there is no consensus on what is the right thing to do.

During the summer in Ireland, most experts agree that SPF 30 is high enough, unless it's unusually sunny. However, SPF 50+ should be forcibly handed to the whole of Ireland at the airport when they go on a sun holiday. Perhaps police could patrol the Costas and the Canaries looking for Irish people sweating in the sun and confiscate their socks and sandals as punishment? And anyone with sensitive skin, especially rosacea sufferers, should always sunscreen themselves to this level if there's any chance of a shot of sunshine – anything less might result in hot flushing misery.

The best sunscreens

It actually doesn't matter what price range you go for when it comes to body sunscreens once they work. A Which? report tested fifteen popular sunscreens and found that price is no indication of quality. Aldi's own-brand sunscreen passed with flying colours, as did Nivea Sun Moisturising Sun Lotion and Boots Soltan Dry Touch Suncare Lotion.

Facial sunscreens are a little different as other factors come into play, like sensitivity, eye stingy-ness, compatibility with make-up, the horror of Ghost Face and so on. All sound trivial compared with cancer, but they are enough to create a minefield of confusion and cause a lot of people not to bother with facial sunscreen.

A combination of physical sunblock (look out for zinc oxide and titanium dioxide in the ingredient list) and a chemical sunblock with UVA and UVB protection (this is combination is known as 'broad spectrum' sunscreen) is what most sunscreens provide. A warning though: too much physical sunblock in the formula will give you Ghost Face, particularly in flash photography, and super-pale Ghost Face is something to be avoided at all costs. If your sunscreen has high levels of physical sunblock, you'll still possess the pale and unholy look of the undead, no matter how much you rub, as these ingredients work by reflecting sunlight off the face. Great for goths and emos, not so much for the rest of us.

To counter instances of this frightening happenstance, throw a séance and summon forth an entity to banish it forever. Alternatively, use a chemical sunscreen or one that's tinted to counteract Ghost Face. If magnesium is added to the sunscreen formula, it cancels out the Ghost Face effect; Boots Soltan Once Face Moisturising Suncare Cream does this and that makes it a good choice.

Clinique City Block Daily Face Protector has been around for an age and it's still one of the best physical sunscreens out there. We are also fans of the moisturising Clarins Sun Wrinkle Control Cream for Face SPF 50+ and Kiehl's Ultra Light Daily UV Defence SPF 50, which provides a great base for make-up.

Shiseido Urban Environment UV Protection Cream Plus SPF 50 is another facial sunscreen we love very much. Moisturising and a perfect base for foundation (it's matte and non-greasy), this cream hydrates and removes easily with a normal cleanser. Another high-spectrum favourite is Mac Prep+Prime Face Protect Lotion SPF 50.

Aldi Lacura UVA and UVB Moisturising Sun Lotion SPF 30 is water-resistant (neither sweat nor tears are getting through this stuff) and it contains green tea and vitamin E. The Aldi broad spectrum creams have been independently tested by Which? and are guaranteed to protect against sun damage just as well as pricier brands.

Oh – and don't make the classic mistake of thinking that because you've used a moisturiser with an SPF 15 and a foundation with SPF 10, you're wearing a combined total of SPF 25. You're not – you're only protected to the level of SPF 15. Sunscreen maths is mean like that.

Beauty tip: Sunscreen and moisturiser

Always put your sunscreen on over your moisturiser.

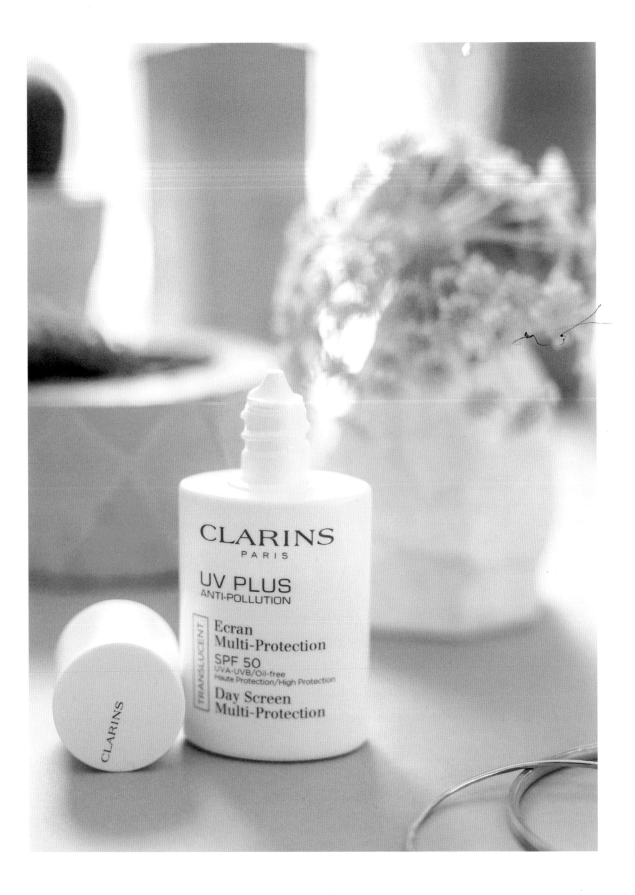

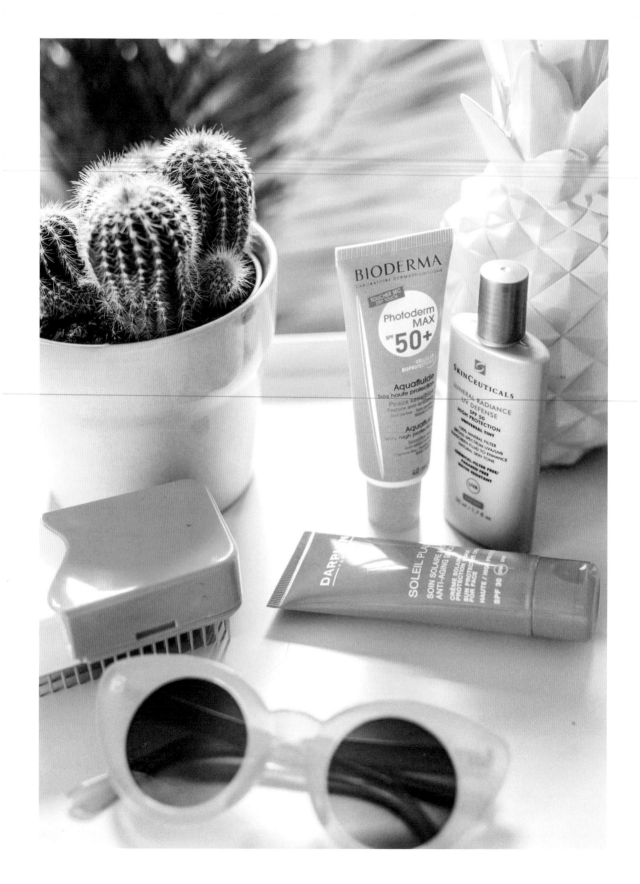

Beauty tip: Extreme sunscreen sensitivity

If you have suffered for years with what you believe is an intense reaction to the sun and you dread sunny weather and the heat of holidays abroad, it may be that those outbreaks of prickly heat and rashes and your need to take antihistamines to calm your face are all be down to your sunscreen and not the heat at all.

Irritation, weeping, puffed-up eyes and acute sensitivity are a source of extreme frustration when they occur but this problem can be solved with the right sunscreen. You need to pick one with more physical blockers than chemical ones because it is chemical blockers that tend to cause extreme reactions. A new sunscreen might quite literally change your life – SkinCeuticals Mineral Radiance UV Defense SPF 50 has a 100% mineral base that makes sure even the most sensitive facial skin can be protected and the tinted formula evens out skin tone too. Clarins UV Plus Anti-Pollution is so good that many users are so attached that they will never choose another sunscreen, even though it comes in the teeniest bottle ever. Avène Very High Protection Mineral Cream SPF 50 is another nice solution for those who like a touch of tint along with their sun protection. Its tinted formula means you won't get Ghost Face, even though it only contains mineral blockers. And Ultrasun Professional Protection·Face SPF 50 is a solid fix for holidays when particularly high sun protection is needed. It's free from oils and scent, which cuts down on the risk of allergy.

Beauty decoded: Alphabet Creams and SPF

This is one of the (probably the only) times that Alphabet Creams (page 143) should come into their own, offering sun protection and decent coverage. Unfortunately, this is so far from the case that sun protection was left on the floor beside the Alphabet Cream case and was never even packed. So while BB, CC, DD, EE and WTF* creams should all act to give you decent sun protection, glow, foundationy coverage and all that jazz, not all of them do, making informed comparison impossible. Their sun protection capabilities range from the very good to the absolutely useless, so make sure you check the label carefully.

Lancôme Soleil Bronzer Smoothing Protective BB Cream SPF 50 is a winner when you don't want to bother with foundation and sunscreen. When it's hot, no one wants a faceful of make-up sliding off their face and this BB cream gives you sun protection and complexion-enhancing in one. Powerful filters shield skin from the sun while the tinted formula conceals imperfections and blemishes. Estée Lauder Enlighten EE Skintone Corrector and YSL Forever Light Creator CC Cream are also favourites of ours.

*WTF doesn't exist. We just made that up. But you see where we're going with it.

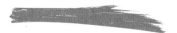

CHAPTER 8
· SKIN CHALLENGES ·

Years ago when Aisling was newly promoted in the early stages of her job, she had to make a presentation to another branch of the company on new innovations that had been made. A practice run-through with her more experienced colleagues was going well until she got to the slide labelled 'Problems', which discussed the, well, problems that had occurred during the changes. Immediately, she was interrupted. 'No, no, not problems, never problems! Challenges. Concerns. That's how we manage this.'

While at the time she thought this was all a bit OTT and office-speak the likes of which Ricky Gervais would be proud of, they had a point.

The change in terminology from 'problems' to 'challenges' did in fact minimise the troublesome factors, transforming them from insurmountable difficulties into stages that could be overcome. So that's what we're going to do with all these skincare issues: minimise them by treating them as simple concerns that can be overcome using tried-and-tested methods.

From adult acne to rosacea and hyperpigmentation, let's see how we can fire those 'challenges' on a rocket to the heart of the boiling sun, dust ourselves down and continue on with our lives.

Adult acne

Cursing is perfectly permissible when talking about acne, especially adult acne, so we'll say right off the bat that it's a bastard of a thing to happen. Most of us assumed spots would be left behind in our teens, along with hopes that the school would burn down in the night and the horrible possibility that we might die a virgin. Hopefully the virginity bit is a distant memory (and if it isn't, we're sorry we can't help – it isn't that kind of book), but the acne part may only be just beginning.

Men don't usually go through an adult acne crisis as their hormones settle down post-puberty, leaving them to sail through life with zero hormonal ups and downs and thus with much better skin than women. Not only is men's skin usually blemish-free, it is also thicker and oiler, which generally means less wrinkles. And not to labour a feminist point, but men don't generally give a toss about their wrinkles anyway because they simply are not under the same sort of pressure that women are to look youthful.

Anywaaaay *both sigh heavily* let's not bother discussing the patriarchy here – we'll get back to adult acne instead. For many women, the spectre of spots and full-on acne remains over the course of our lives and can appear suddenly without any warning even if you've had perfectly behaved skin all your life. It is a surprisingly common condition and we can thank our damned hormones for that.

Think about it: a woman's hormones go through so many changes and surges, among them puberty, going on the pill, coming off the pill, pregnancy, perimenopause and menopause. Add to that any medical conditions such as polycystic ovary syndrome and you've got many, many triggers for acne. Really, when you think about it, your whole life is basically a potential acne trigger and for some reason, turning forty seems to put you right in the danger zone.

It's nothing short of desperate to have to deal with breakouts in your thirties, forties and beyond, but the positive part of all this is that it is very easy to treat adult acne and it is often the cheaper products that are most effective. Although our natural impulse when faced with a crop of spots is to try and blast them into the stratosphere, it is really important to steer clear of the caustic products aimed at the teen acne market. They are

It is a surprisingly common condition and we can thank our damned hormones for that.

Cleansers and toners laden with alcohol might dry out the spot and give you ostensibly speedy results, but they also dehydrate the surrounding skin, possibly leave you with scarring, and don't tackle the long-term problem.

far too harsh for anyone to use, particularly on thirty-, forty- and fifty-something skin that is much thinner and often less oily – and in fact those alcohol-laden products are far too harsh even for teen skin.

Treating adult acne is all about the cleansing. Laura is an adult acne veteran and she now has the most perfect skin anyone could hope to have. She cleared up her acne with a strict regime that centres around double cleansing, liquid toners/exfoliants, masks and serums. Although this might seem like a lot of work, it really isn't: we're talking about ten minutes per night max. You'll get addicted to the feeling of your skin as it clears, you'll look and feel so much more confident and you'll have put in place a long-term solution to solve your skin challenges. (As well as changing her skincare routine, Laura also went to her doctor about her acne. The pill was an element in managing the hormonal aspects of her acne, as acne is often both hormonal and bacterial. We suggest visiting your GP to diagnose the type of acne.)

Don't go for the quick fix is our advice. Cleansers and toners laden with alcohol might dry out your spots and give you ostensibly speedy results, but they also dehydrate the surrounding skin, possibly leave you with scarring, and don't tackle the long-term problem. The spots will keep on returning and you'll keep on feeling miserable.

BHAs are your saviour (see page 20) so zone in on anything with salicylic acid in the ingredient list, such as Murad Clarifying Cleanser, Bioderma Sébium Pore Refiner Corrective Concentrate, Úna Brennan Super Facialist Salicylic Acid Anti-Blemish Purifying Cleansing Wash (try the mask in this range as well for extra pore-clearing benefits), Garnier PureActive Anti-Blackhead Deep Pore Wash and Avène Cleanance K. Really step it up a notch if you want to spend a little more with Estée Lauder Idealist Dual Action Refinishing Treatment, which is a bit of a wonder in the pore-clearing stakes.

Funnily enough, the same ingredient, salicylic acid, is used to unblock and free ingrown hairs that cause nasty lumps and bumps after waxing and epilating by dissolving away dead skin and clearing out the pores. If you already have wipes that you use to free those hairs, you'll find that they work just as well on your face – try Waxperts Ingrown Hair Pads or Bliss Ingrown Eliminating Pads. It sounds completely whack but it works just as well whether it's your ladygarden area or your chin. Let's just call salicylic acid an equal opportunities pore unblocker. Gentle cleansers like those from Aveeno, Avène or Simple are ideal. Wash your face twice a day with warm water and use your fingers to massage in the cleanser. Be gentle as you don't want to rub and scrub, just dissolve away dirt and grease. While you're at

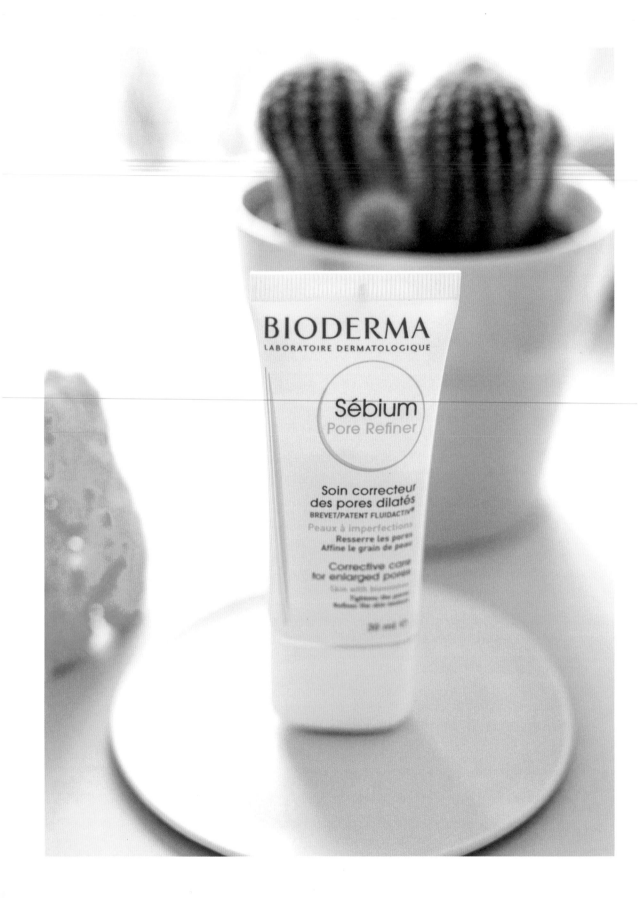

it, throw your scrubby exfoliator in the bin as anything with 'beads' or gritty 'bits', like apricot kernels, in it will only aggravate everything. How that stuff is still being made is beyond us.

Instead follow up your cleanser with a low-level salicylic or glycolic acid toner or liquid exfoliator. This will unclog pores, sweep away dead skin cells and won't over-dry or aggravate your skin. Clarins Gentle Exfoliator Brightening Toner is a good one. If you don't want to get into the palaver of using a separate toner, use something quick like Nip+Fab Glycolic Fix Exfoliating Facial Pads.

If you use a cleanser with salicylic, lactic or gly-colic acid already included, like Úna Brennan

Super Facialist Salicylic Acid Anti-Blemish Purifying Cleansing Wash, you might find you can dispense with toner altogether. Just watch out for cleansers that promise to 'mattify' or control shine – they are often loaded with alcohol or other drying agents.

If at-home methods have not produced the results you were hoping for, there is no need for despair. Dermatologists have a box of tricks at their disposal to calm even the most stubborn acne. From prescribed medicine to topical preparations, including retinol, or a course of laser or IPL to treat scar damage or a particularly bad outbreak, they will be able to get those lumps and bumps under control.

If at-home methods have not produced the results you were hoping for, there is no need for despair. Dermatologists have a box of tricks at their disposal to calm even the most stubborn acne.

Age spots and hyperpigmentation

The term 'liver spots' always puts us in mind of a toothless crone dwelling in her ginger-bread house, grasping children in her mottled, bony claws, all the better to boil them up in her cauldron. Obviously we read too many spooky fairy tales as youngsters but even so, you can imagine how delighted Aisling was to find dark patches appearing on her face before she was thirty-five.

She has two dark patches on each cheek-bone due to sun damage and in the last

couple of years regular make-up hadn't a hope of disguising them. So who better than to try out all the topical treatments out there to fade dark spots and find out if they actually worked and weren't all talk and no trousers? She decided to try all the things (yes, all of them) to discover the best way to fade the patches, and hopefully erase them all together. It turns out that there are literally dozens of ingredients to lighten skin discolouration, and most of them are natur-ally occurring. Some of them would in fact be a delicious addition to the gingerbread house: liquorice features prominently as a lightening ingredient.

The way in which these brighteners work is quite simple. They gently and chemically remove dead skin cells so that those that are stained and discoloured are gradually lifted away. Gradual really is the name of the game here though, as there are no quick fixes with at-home treatments. If you are desperate for the patches to be gone instantly, you'll need to book into a dermatologist for a course of laser treatment. Otherwise you are looking at a timeline of four to six weeks. At least.

If you're looking for a tried and trusted serum that includes tons of skin-brightening goodness, try Clinique Even Better Clinical Dark Spot Corrector, Indeed Labs Pepta-bright Even Skin Tone Enhancer and Neostrata Skin Brightener. Dermalogica C-12 Pure Bright Serum is great for sloughing off dead skin cells and evening out skin tone.

Philosophy No Reason To Hide Multi-Imperfection Transforming Serum is another serum to add to the arsenal of anti-hyperpigmentation products. It feels silky and hydrating and the powerhouse skin-brightening ingredient list gets the thumbs up. SkinCeuticals Advanced Pigment Corrector is an absolute super-strength favourite. If your dark spots don't run shrieking at the sight of these creams, then we will be amazed.

While these products will work on any skin tone, if you want a more targeted approach,

Lancôme DreamTone Ultimate Dark Spot Corrector, available in three custom formulations for black, Asian and white skin tones, is the one to try. A more reasonably priced alternative that always gets good feedback is Garnier Skin Renew Dark Spot Corrector.

If you already use a chemical or liquid toner, then you are ahead of the game, particularly if contains an AHA like glycolic or lactic acid. Vitamin C is also a great pigmentation shifter and while fizzing a Berocca on your face might not have the same result (although, who knows … *hurries to try*), a skin brightener containing it will help to clear your skin.

One caveat: only use these products at night because they cause your skin to become sensitive to the sun.

It is also important to remember that even though you may have cleared up the dark patches, they are very likely to reappear from time to time. Every time she goes on a sun holiday, despite using SPF 50, Aisling knows when she returns home she will probably have to tackle the hyperpigmentation issue all over again, but the marks are never that noticeable and quickly fade.

Beauty decoded: Pregnancy mask

Melasma is a variation of hyperpigmentation that is caused by changing hormone levels during pregnancy and leads to skin darkening and patchy colouring. The good news is that it usually leaves when the baby arrives.

Blackheads

Okay. You've rubbed, you've scrubbed – even though we begged you not to – and you've tried every damn method of squeezing and used so many horrible antiseptic smelling lotions and still those blackheads won't shift. You can practically give them names because they've lived on your nose for as long as you can remember and make-up only accentuates those blocked pores and rough skin.

They seem to have a half-life of plutonium – as soon as they're gone they come back again. They are basically the Terminator of the acne world.

However, we're going to get all Sarah Connor on them right now. I'll be back? I don't think so.

Skin is constantly regenerating and in a perfect world, dead skin cells would slither off like the skin of a snake, leaving you to emerge from a cocoon, regenerated with fresh, soft, gleaming skin. But snakes have a much better deal than us: a lot of our dead skin cells 'glue' themselves to new skin and plug up our pores. If hair follicles get blocked with dead skin and excess oil, they form blackheads. Quite often, no matter how many times they are squeezed, they continue to fill up. Our tried and tested method for dealing with blackheads takes just two easy steps: the first is to get rid of the gunk in your pores and the second is to keep it from filling up again.

If you have a lot of blockage, the first thing you might consider is getting them professionally extracted rather than poking and prodding yourself, which could cause scarring and infection. This involves a lot of squeezing, wiping guckage off onto tissues and a strong-stomached therapist – but don't worry, you don't have anything they haven't dealt with before. It also feels like your nose is actually being broken in half, but it is so worth it.

One of the simplest ways to dissolve the gunk is to use a regular dose of BHA. There are loads of different AHAs around, such as lactic and glycolic acids but salicylic acid is the only BHA (see page 20 for more). While AHAs are water-based and work on the surface of skin, salicylic acid goes one step further: it gets in underneath the pores to shift the blockage from the inside. It's very difficult for any ingredient to penetrate the skin's barrier (the skin is, after all, designed to keep things out and will repel most ingredients). But salicylic acid is able to dive right to the bottom of pores because it is oil-soluble and better able to penetrate oil-filled pores. Regular use will stop the pores from refilling too.

Bioré Blemish Fighting Ice Cleanser, which has 2% salicylic acid, works without harshness and the price point is perfect for the younger market. Nip+Fab Dragon's Blood Fix Cleansing Pads provide a quick and easy fix. When you want to bring in the big guns, a face mask infused with salicylic will work wonders; use Origins Out of Trouble 10 Minute Mask to Rescue Problem Skin to kickstart a declogging regime. Lots of moisturisers also contain the magic salicylic acid; Olay Total Effects 7-in-1 Anti-Ageing Blemish Care Moisturiser is one for the over-thirty-fives.

And now, just one last piece of wisdom to impart. Never Google 'blackhead extraction' and watch the videos on YouTube. We know this will make many of you rush immediately to the internet, but don't say we didn't warn you.

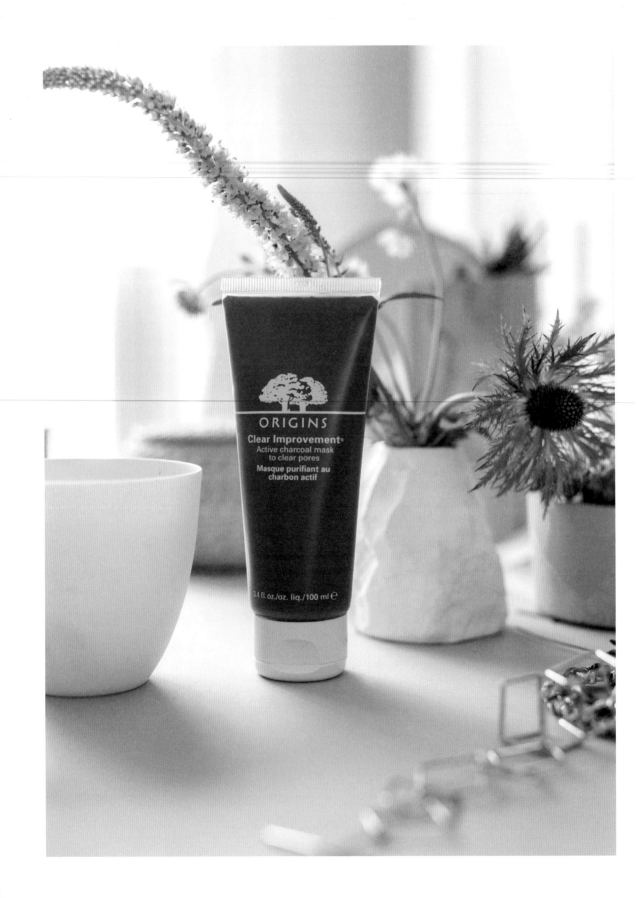

Dehydrated skin

Skin loses moisture as we age, but dehydrated skin can strike at any age, especially during the winter as we crank up the heating and spend more time inside in dry, over-heated environments. Harsh weather, bitter cold and the freezing wind we battle with during the winter months all add to this perfect storm of attack against the skin's barrier system.

For Aisling, the first warning sign that her skin is shrivelling up quicker than a sun-dried tomato is when the skin at the bridge of her nose gets rough and flaky. This leads to nasty little dehydration lines under the eyes and makes her skin look dull and rough.

To combat dehydrated skin, cleansing with gentle, creamy cleansers is a must. Exfoliation and using a good facial oil to trap moisture in dry and dehydrated skin work really well and serums and moisturisers with hyaluronic acid, niacin and glycerin also are a godsend.

DRY AND DEHYDRATED

Dry skin doesn't produce enough oil. Dehydrated skin lacks water, which has been sucked out by anything from natural ageing to environmental conditions (that radiator set too high, the air con in the office, the bitter weather outside). So to combat this quick route to instant fine lines, you'll need to add both water and oil to your skin. Up your moisturising game by choosing a good hydrating serum or face mask to put that moisture back into your skin, exfoliate properly to get rid of dead skin cells so that moisture can penetrate new skin effectively and if you have been using moisturiser alone up to now, add in an oil to see a difference almost overnight.

Your skin is crying out for oil – give it lashings. Dry and dehydrated skin drinks up facial oils and it only takes a couple of drops morning and night to make a real difference. If you find your skin greedily drinks up those couple of drops recommended on the label, then give it as much as it needs. It should feel supple and comfortable.

Mix a rich moisturiser with the oil to seal in it in, keeping all that moisture locked in and your skin protected and soft. At night, you can try out sleeping masks and overnight gel masks. It only takes a few days to see results and you'll be amazed at the improvement.

OILY AND DEHYDRATED

It is a misconception that only dry skin becomes dehydrated. While oily skin may be producing bucket-loads of sebum, it can dehydrate by losing moisture in just the same way that dry skin does – central heating and harsh weather once more being the main culprit for dried-out skin. Although it seems like a contradiction, oily skin needs lots of moisture if you feel it getting tight or flaky or if your foundation clings to dry bits of your face and slides off other parts.

Exfoliate gently and use a good serum under your oil-free moisturiser to prevent causing more grease than the fryers in Borzas on a Friday night. Yon-ka Hydra No1 Serum, Indeed Labs Hyaluron Moisture Booster or Caudalie Vinosource S.O.S. Thirst Quenching Serum are ideal for this skin type. If you'd like to add an oil, use a 'drier' type, such L'Oréal Age Perfect Extraordinary Facial Oil.

Stay far, far away from harsh foaming face-washes and cleansers and anything with a lot of alcohol in its ingredients, as these will only cause further misery. This goes for all skin types – it's bitter outside, you want to cocoon and soothe inside.

Bargain beauty: Coconut oil and Vaseline

Don't swoon in shock – this is a brilliant way to deeply moisturise your skin. Use coconut oil after cleansing and seal it in with Vaseline at night. Just remember to cleanse it off well in the morning so that your morning skincare can penetrate and work during the day. If you want to spend some money, invest in Elizabeth Arden Eight Hour Cream Skin Protectant or Rodial Glam Balm Multi as they provide a similar barrier that nothing will get through, making sure all your delicious serum, oil and moisturiser stay close to your phizog all night.

Bargain beauty: Bikini wipes

You know those wipes that prevent ingrown hairs on your legs and bikini areas? Well, they use the same BHA as skincare products and also dissolve spots and blackheads. Try ingrown hair wipes from Waxperts or Bliss.

DEHYDRATED LIMBS

Don't forget about body skin either – it's just as prone to the shrivel and a good rich night treatment will do it the world of good. Ever heard of dandruff legs? That's our tasteful term for what happens when those limbs are stuffed into tights and jeans for the whole winter without a lick of moisture. Whether you shave them or not when no one is going to see them is your business, but we can bet most of you are not too bothered about keeping them smooth and gleaming during the bleak winter months, hence the specks of skin showing up on your black opaques.

It's okay, we've all been there. A good exfoliation and lashings of a thick body cream, or preferably body butter, over the course of a few days will get you back on track. Whether you choose to shave or wax those legs as well is definitely a feminist issue, so we'll leave that decision completely up to you.

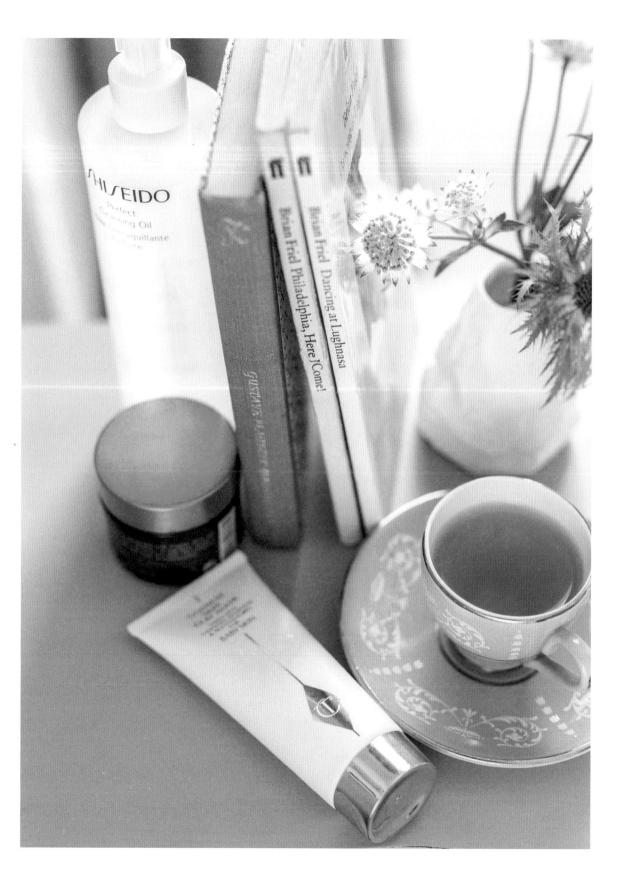

Mature skin

For the sake of providing some kind of indicator of what we mean when we talk about mature skin, we'll say it's from the age of fifty-plus. Of course, as with all things to do with the human body, some people's skin begins to act in a mature fashion much earlier, sensibly wanting to start a pension and staying in its slippers on weeknights, while its immature counterparts get away with partying 'til dawn for much longer without a line on their faces.

Contrary to popular opinion, genetics only has a small part to play in skin ageing: 20% of how your skin looks is genetic while the other 80% is down to how you live and how you've treated it. So sun damage, general health, hormones, smoking and environmental issues have a huge part to play in healthy-looking skin.

Reading the list of things that happen to mature skin is enough to make you want to stick your head in the oven, so we'll just briefly gloss over this part and then quickly leap to all the wonderful treats and practical pro-ageing steps you can take to make sure your skin looks as great as humanly possible. (Forever.)

So gloss off now if you don't want to read the list of horrors, which includes loss of collagen, elastin, bigger pores, dryness, sagging, loss of firmness and plumpness, jowls, crepe neck and crepey eyes.

Well you know what we say to that? Bah. And we also say: Helen Mirren.

Inside every woman is a beautiful, sexier-with-every-year-that-passes Helen Mirren.

And with good attention to your skincare routine and lots of time for yourself (because let's face it, you deserve it after reading that depressing list), you will find that your skin once again glows with health and looks more radiant.

Diagnosing yourself with mature or maturing skin is not the desperate thing it may sound. On the contrary, it's the excuse, nay reason, to indulge in the richest creams and the most luxurious oils and to have a bit of a splurge on a brand you've always wanted to try, after you tried out a sample first of course.

At birth our skin cells are composed of about 75% water, which declines to around 50% as we grow older. This is the reason mature skin can look saggy and draggy: it's programmed to dehydrate naturally. We've all heard the mantra about rehydrating from within with eight glasses of water a day but to be honest, the jury is still out on how effective that really is. The skin on the neck and hands and under the eyes are especially thin, with less fat padding underneath them, so no amount of water imbibing is going to really affect them. But we need to get some water back into those skin cells, even if only temporarily, and moisturise to the max to make skin gleam, firm up those jowls and make the skin look smoother and pores appear smaller. All of this is possible.

But there is one thing you must do first.

It's time to brave the depths of the bathroom cabinet. Take an honest look at the products you are using at the moment. Are you still using that skin cream you used in your thirties and wondering why it doesn't work anymore? Your skin has changed and you might have to adjust your products to stay looking great – unless you are Joanna Lumley, of course, who has used Astral Cream for her entire life and sees no reason to change. If you too feel your products work, then stick with them.

Sadly most of us are not Joanna Lumley so it might be time for a few old reliables to hit the bin. There is no time like the present to assess what lurks within. One good way to tell if something doesn't suit your skin is to do the dust test: if it's covered in a generous coating, then you are never going to use it. Another good way to judge if something might just possibly be past its use by date – and we're going out on a limb here – is if you spy the price tag is in Irish pounds. Don't break your heart laughing – we've heard worse stories than this. In fact, we wouldn't be surprised if one of our mothers still had a jar of some revolting 'skin food' priced in shillings.

Don't hang on to it 'just in case'. You hate it. It doesn't work.

Say goodbye.

Do it. Do it now.

Beauty tip: Six ways to keep mature skin looking great

It's time to learn to read the ingredients on the packaging of your pro-ageing moisturiser or serum to make sure the contents are actually going to help firm and moisturise your skin and not just make ridiculous over-the-top promises. And remember, the further down the list of ingredients something is, the less of it there actually is in the product.

USE MOISTURISERS WITH COLLAGEN, ELASTIN AND NIACIN

Although many pro-ageing products swear on their granny's life that the proteins, peptides, collagen and elastin contained in their creams will instantly youthalise you 'from within', they are far too large to get through the skin. Don't write them off entirely though, as they're great moisturisers and can help make the skin more supple and reduce the look of fine lines and wrinkles.

AHAS, RETINOL AND VITAMIN C IN MOISTURISER ARE ALL GOOD

You should also try pro-ageing moisturisers that contain these ingredients, as they help to lift the top layer of dead skin cells, reducing the appearance of fine lines, and may also stimulate collagen production. Retinol reduces wrinkles and repairs sun damage. Vitamin C can increase collagen production and, amazingly enough, gives some protection from UV rays. It has been proven that a combination of antioxidants in a product is far better than one on its own so look for quality brands with these ingredients.

USE A GENTLE LIQUID/CHEMICAL TONER OR ESSENCE

A lot of older women we speak to, particularly those with post-menopausal skin, tell us that they don't exfoliate. When we ask them why, they tell us that their skin is too dry or that it is too delicate. And it's true, mature skin is far too fragile to use scratchy scrubs with 'bits' like apricot kernels because they will tear the face off you and could lead to broken veins. Actually, everyone's skin is too delicate to use this kind of scrub.

But you do need to exfoliate because as cell turnover decreases with age, all that old dead skin will remain 'glued' to your face unless it is sloughed off. Softly, softly does it, and sometimes a facecloth is all you will need to gently exfoliate if you don't want to chance even the gentlest of AHAs.

USE SERUMS AND MOISTURISERS WITH HYALURONIC ACID AND GLYCERIN

Although it occurs naturally in the body anyway, the use of hyaluronic acid in skincare has really taken off and with good reason. It is a humectant that absorbs up to 1,200 times its own weight in water from the atmosphere and uses this water to plump up skin, fill in fine lines and make skin look fresher. There is no phoney science here: this stuff works immediately and is perfect for mature skin, especially when incorporated with antioxidant ingredients. Getting it injected directly into

your wrinkles is even better, but we'll leave that up to you.

Glycerin is another humectant and it is one of the most common ingredients around because it is cheap and works well to help keep skin moisturised and soft, preventing dryness, so look out for moisturisers and serums with these magic agents.

DON'T STRESS ABOUT YOUR WEIGHT

We've all heard the saying 'figure over face' and unless you are willing to invest in fat plumping injections and fillers, don't worry about your weight as you get older. Of course, some of us are naturally very slim so there's not much we can do about this. Fat loss can unfortunately age facial features and leads to sagging and loss of firmness. A bit of weight plumps out your skin and keeps it looking healthy, so that bit of extra weight you stress about may do you good.

USE SUNSCREEN

Unfortunately, age means that you don't have the collagen and elastin reserves in your skin or the ability to regenerate them that you once did. This means that it is doubly important that you protect your skin from the effects of the sun as it simply can't renew the damage.

A bit of weight plumps out your skin and keeps it looking healthy, so that bit of extra weight you stress about may do you good.

Period Face

You start crying at ads on television, being cut up by a White Van Man at the traffic lights sends you into a fit of road rage of ridiculous proportions and God help anyone who jumps in front of you in the queue at the supermarket. Where, for some reason, your basket is loaded up with chocolate and crisps, even though you don't really remember putting them in there.

The only things that don't annoy you are your cat or dog, and even they are getting on your nerves just a little bit with their constant adoration.

Sure enough, the next morning you wake up with the feeling that a knife is scraping your womb out from the inside and cramps that feel like an alien is about to burst out of you any second.

To compound the misery, a quick glance in the mirror confirms that you do indeed have Period Face to go along with all this joy. Spots, breakouts and a puffy face are all symptoms of the dreaded Period Face, yet another thing that makes Mother Nature's monthly gift such a massive pain in the hoop. And worse still, the spots tend to be the sore kind, lining up along the jawline or around the mouth, refusing to come to a head and lurking in painful, cyst-like misery.

Your skin is probably over-producing oil as your hormones rage, and for that reason it is worth trying a few different products to sort out the symptoms.

Use calming and soothing skincare. Now is not the time for rubbing and scrubbing and using harsh products or creams with strong fragrance. A nice balm or cream cleanser will help to soothe skin. Continue the kid gloves treatment by using a light moisturiser. Dermalogica Active Moist is good as is Simple Light Moisturiser.

Don't use harsh or caustic products on the spots even though you are dying to. Calming them down with a facial oil like Trilogy Certified Organic Rosehip Oil means any scarring will be lessened and investing in a good concealer will probably mean that you are the only person who will notice your minor eruptions.

We're all different. Some people find their skin actually clears up during their period, especially if they're on the pill. If you get pale, washed-out and drained-looking, then brightening make-up will be your saving grace. These are the days to turn to CC creams under make-up and luminous powder and blush. Charlotte Tilbury Wonder Glow is a good example of a CC-esque brightener that mixes with your foundation to give your skin a pick me up.

Some of us feel that our face puffs up so much that our eyes look like beady holes sunk into the heel of a batch loaf (which, incidentally, you may feel like eating in its entirety to cheer yourself up). Cooling and calming are the name of the game here, particularly around the eyes. A good cooling eye cream to depuff will help tremendously. Garnier Skin Renew Anti-Dark-Circle Roller and Estée Lauder Idealist Cooling Eye Illuminator (which has a brilliant stone-cold applicator) are great choices, and they also contain light concealers that stop eyes looking like sinkholes.

Now don't rip the heads off us, but the power of a cup of tea, a bar of Dairy Milk and two Nurofen should never be underestimated either.

Radiator Face

Winter brings horrible challenges for your skin as it struggles to battle with both the elements outside and the artificial climate indoors. If you spend most of the stormy weather inside with the central heating turned up all the way to 11, chances are you suffer from a nice dose of Radiator Face every year.

Nothing sucks the moisture out of skin like the dry air of central heating, and harsh weather does skin no favours either. Plunging your skin into a super-heated environment, such as the sitting room, when seconds earlier you were being assaulted by freezing winds is no good for your poor skin. The result is a phisog drier than the Sahara.

Obviously, the best way to cope with this winter onslaught is to stay indoors 24/7, stroking kittens, sipping hot chocolate beside a roaring fire and watching Netflix while one of the blokes from *Magic Mike XXL* rubs your feet. But just in case this doesn't happen, here's the best way to look after your delicate visage.

Start off with the basics. Use a cleanser that's gentle and actually moisturises as it cleans – try a cream- or an oil-based cleanser. Secondly, make sure to gently exfoliate: if your skin is clogged, it won't be receptive to moisturiser.

Serum is the saviour of distressed skin. Think of it as concentrated moisture and nutrients, and look for products with hyaluronic acid in the ingredient list. This is your key weapon in the fight against Radiator Face and will keep that precious moisture in your skin where it belongs.

Don't think your skin is protected just because it's oily: read the 'Oily and dehydrated' section on p83 and you'll see that it most definitely isn't.

Make your night moisturisers more hydrating by mixing them with a couple of drops of any facial oil (We like Liz Earle and Kinvara) and you'll emerge from under the duvet more fresh-faced in the morning. Or go one better and use a hydrating mask such as Indeed Labs Hydraluron Boosting Masks, which is hyaluronic acid-rich, the cult Vitamin E Sink-In Moisture Mask from The Body Shop or Nars Aqua Gel Luminous Mask, which can all be left overnight for softer, smoother skin.

So let the wind howl – your skin will be hydrated and cared for, no matter how high you turn up those rads.

Serum is the saviour of distressed skin. Think of it as concentrated moisture and nutrients, and look for products with hyaluronic acid in the ingredient list.

Rosacea

It's been called the Curse of the Celts and that moniker is bang on the money. The Irish have the highest incidence of rosacea in the world, with one in ten of us suffering from this uncomfortable and embarrassing problem. Rosacea sufferers can blame their fair, photosensitive skin and the harsh Irish weather for that. Not only does it leave sufferers red of face, it can also cause them to develop 'porter nose': a swollen and red snoz that unfairly makes everyone think the victim is a mad alcoholic and can lead to much sniggering and derision. There's no use in protesting that your alcohol intake consists solely of a Baileys at Christmas, because Irish people, being the suspicious and piss-taking lot we are, will not believe you.

It's a horrid state of affairs.

MILDER CASES OF ROSACEA

If you've got mild rosacea, the chances are you don't know. Most people with mild facial redness just get on with things and don't realise there is anything they can do to prevent the hot flushing.

Stress makes it worse so naturally – naturally – this is a condition that tends to make its presence known at the most inconvenient times. On a first date, say, or the morning of your daughter's wedding or just before that interview for the job of your dreams.

So if a few sips of alcohol, a stress-filled day or a shot of sunshine are enough to transform your cheeks and nose into a burning, red, irritable monster mask with the texture of wood-chip wallpaper, then it's more than likely you've got rosacea. You've got one of the most extreme manifestations of sensitive skin. Actually, it shouldn't be called 'sensitive', as if its feelings have been hurt. It should be called bloody bad-tempered, because that's what it is.

Lashings of high-factor sunscreen are an absolute must. In fact, the rosacea-prone shouldn't step outside without an SPF 50 – even on a normal day, let alone the dizzying heights of the Irish 'summer' – and it's probably worth investing in some lovely hats to keep even more of the sun off your face.

Keep your skincare as natural as possible by avoiding additives, chemicals, fragrance and alcohol. Find your triggers and avoid them, even though sadly they seem to be some of the ones that make life fun: alcohol, spicy food and aromatic ingredients can spark off an attack of the dreaded red.

Keep it simple and don't mess with your skin too much. Leave the glycolic acids and peels to others and the trying out of new whizz-bang fabulous-sounding treatments to people with stronger skin. You just want everything to calm the hell down. Practical products that relieve irritation and inflammation, improve the skin's barrier for long-term relief and smooth the surface of the skin are what we're after. It's time to sort out that bad-tempered skin once and for all.

Silcock's Base is one of the best, cheapest and

most moisturising ways to remove make-up and soothe skin. It might block your pores though, so if you would like a more thorough wash, Cetaphil Gentle Skin Cleanser is non-drying, pH-neutral and gentle, and won't strip the skin of comforting natural oils. A bonus: it will efficiently dispatch an entire face of make-up down the plug hole. The packaging is refreshingly unisex and will appeal to those who want to quickly wash up and move on with their day. If you suffer from flaky or 'scaly' skin, Bioderma Sensibio DS+ Purifying, Soothing Cleansing Gel works on skin irritants and reddening right at the cleansing stage, while the Dermalogica Ultracalming trio of cleanser, moisturiser and serum gives redness a kick in the pants with its triple threat approach.

The Avène Antirougeurs range has a whole heap of excellent products dedicated to cooling, calming and taking out the sensation and appearance of redness. Bioderma Sensibio AR BB Cream is a nice one to try to not only treat the redness but also to disguise it. It is a light foundation that keeps on soothing skin by improving its barrier function with long-term use. Uriage Roseliane Anti-Redness Cream is another cream that soothes and shields the skin from irritants; take it right down your neck as far as your collarbone or further, depending on how low cut your neckline is. If you're flashing your boobs, that's grand by us – just remember your calming cream along with the tit tape so you don't get that annoying flush beginning to rise up your neck. This is a good rule of thumb for any of the rosacea creams.

If stress tends to kick off your rosacea, there are lots of products out there to help, such as Kiehl's Skin Rescuer. It's been formulated with extract of rosa gallica, which helps to fortify the skin's barrier function. If you find your skin flies into a red rage during periods of stress, this may be the one to calm things right down. It's great for skin that's mad as hell and not going to take it anymore.

Developed by Irish dermatologists, Seavite Organic Seaweed Anti-Ageing Cleanser and Seavite Organic Seaweed Moisturising & Replenishing Face Crème use the therapeutic benefits of West of Ireland seaweed to help rough skin to feel smoother and calms down redness and irritation after the first couple of uses. Another Irish brand, Finca, developed in Dundalk, produces Finca Skin Organics Redness Relief Serum, which is primarily a rosehip oil but contains added ingredients that calm and soothe the dreaded rosacea redness, such as vitamin A and lycopene.

Ren Evercalm Anti-Redness Serum is one we particularly like because of its capillary-strengthening action. Rosacea makes sensitive skin thinner and even more fragile over time, as capillaries in the skin burst and create tiny red thread lines, which makes blushing more noticeable. Ren Evercalm Global Protection Day Cream strengthens capillary walls with natural ingredients and produces a cooling effect. It also has a shot of hyaluronic acid to boost hydration so lash it on under your moisturiser. Darphin Intral Redness Recovery Cream, while pricey, is also excellent.

SEVERE ROSACEA

When rosacea becomes inflamed, with spots that leave marks on the skin, it's time to go pro. The best thing to do with acne rosacea is to take it off to a dermatologist and get it nuked. Seriously, they have access to the best antibiotic creams, IPL treatments and whatever the latest doohickeys are to banish the misery. Please don't suffer with this – it's a miserable condition.

ROSACEA AND MEN

Rosacea tends to strike around the thirty to fifty age ranges but to be honest, it can hit at just about any age. While three times more women than men are affected, men tend to get a more severe type, with the added misery of not being able to use make-up to cover up. Luckily enough, the trend for massive beards, the likes of which haven't been seen since Victorian times, might come in handy for disguising purposes.

You can't grow a beard on your nose though, so a good solution for guys is Dermalogica Redness Relief Primer, which tones down redness while calming the skin. Don't be afraid: although it looks scarily green when it comes out of the tube, it blends perfectly into skin and no one will ever know you're wearing it.

Of course all the other products we've recommended in this section are suitable for men, but we understand that the worry and stress of using something in vaguely ladylike packaging might bring on a dose of redness. Use Cetaphil Gentle Skin Cleanser as a cleanser, Elave Sensitive UV Defence Moisturiser for Men as your moisturising anti-redness product (you might need to add a higher SPF over the top of it) and Avène Antirougeurs Fort Relief Concentrate for Chronic Redness to disguise and calm.

This regime should help considerably and you might not even have to grow a beard. Unless you want to, of course.

When rosacea becomes inflamed, with spots that leave marks on the skin, it's time to go pro. The best thing to do with acne rosacea is to take it off to a dermatologist and get it nuked.

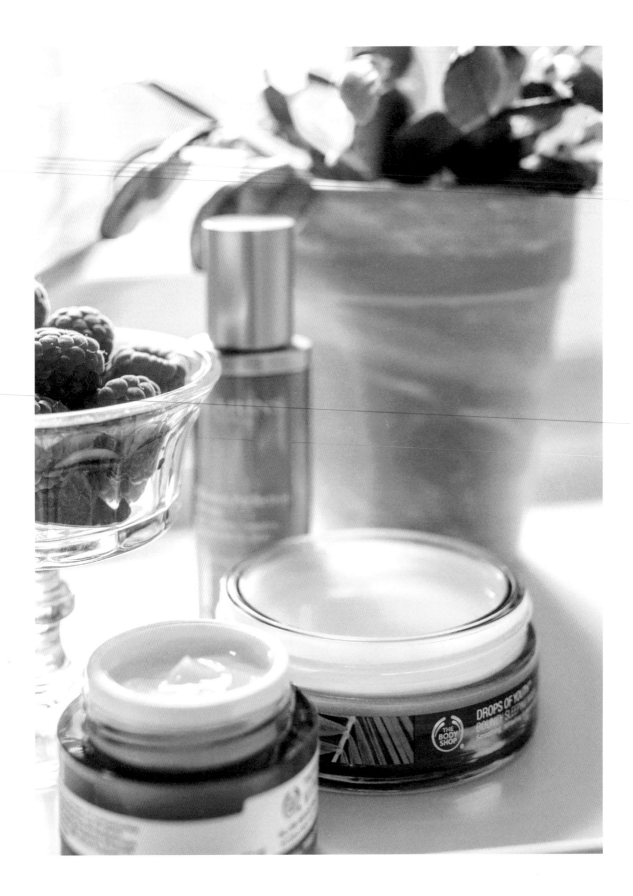

The Detox

By the time January rolls around, many of us are done. Done with boozing, done with endless boxes of Roses, done with late nights and tinsel. It is around about now that we long for the break that is signalled by New Year's Day and the cleanness and sharpness that January signals. A new year is on the way, a new opportunity to renew ourselves and improve whatever we're not happy with. We feel so full of 'tox' that we long to detox, to purge, to plan the diet of all diets and to lose that ten pounds that we feel would make life perfect if we were without.

Should the urge to detox overcome you, no matter the time of year, stop right there. The whole concept of detoxing is a marketing con. Your internal organs and your skin, the biggest organ of elimination, are pretty good at de-toxing all by themselves. In fact, they've been doing it for tens of thousands of years with nary a detox foot patch or green smoothie shake in sight.

The tox will get out all by itself. You might feel saggy and crinkly with lines in places you didn't even know you had places before now but rest assured, this will not be a permanent fixture. Get back to your normal diet, drink all the water you can (before Irish Water has some kind of meltdown and is unable to deliver its only product), and 'eat' as much water as you can in the form of fruits and vegetables.

The urge to detox might leap at you at other times too. If you are having a crisis of any kind – post-holiday, post-three-day-wedding – or if life is being a pain in the ass and giving you no precious me time, you might feel like embarking on some class of torture to purge yourself. Don't.

So you're knackered, you've bags under your eyes that would take you over an airline luggage limit and your skin is as scaly as a dried up fish. There's no need to punish yourself like a 14th-century monk in a hairshirt by doing things like lymphatic drainage and coffee enemas. No, the actions you need to take to make yourself feel like a normal human being again are *nice*.

Naturally, lots of moisture is the answer. Cleanse your face properly, exfoliate, take lovely seaweed baths and then go to town with all those moisturisers and overnight masks you've bought and never finished. Finish everything – except the things so old they have a Switzers sticker on them.

Have a few nights in with a cup of tea, saying 'no' to all those things you don't want to do in a pleasant yet assertive manner. Go to bed early. Don't eat any crap. Watch many boxsets. In fact, boxsets may possibly be the newest and best method of detox.

Follow all the tips in the 'Dehydrated Skin' section (page 83) and you'll be sorted. And if you can find a special offer for a nice salon massage or facial, it will do you the world of good.

CHAPTER 9

· NECK ·

No discussion of the face can realistically occur without including something about the neck.

Ideally we should treat the neck as an extension of the face, but most of us don't bother about it. We rarely think about the fact that it is out and about as much as the face, living life with *joi de vivre* and enjoying both sun holidays and bracing walks in the rain – and it has been doing all of this with thinner skin than the face and with less oil and sweat glands to protect it. Unless you've had a lifelong love affair with polo necks, your skin has been up against the exact same environmental damage as your face.

But don't worry, lots can be done to help the neck area, even if you feel like you may have left it a bit late. Like everything else, prevention is of course better than cure.

SPF really is the magic ingredient here; if you get into the habit of using sun protection on your neck from a young age, you will be filled with neckly gratitude when you get a bit older. Aisling, a child of the 1970s, of course never used sun protection and remembers one particularly bad episode of neck abuse. It was a sunny day in West Cork, the kind of magical day that can only occur in that magical place, and she spent the entire day in a beer garden enjoying drinks and soaking up the sun with nary a tube of sunscreen in sight, while wearing a necklace with a huge butterfly on it. By that night, her whole neck and chesticle area was burned red raw – with the exception of that butterfly shape. A tan tattoo. The shame.

If you're someone who never bothers to moisturise your neck, you're certainly not alone. Very few of us do until we're into our late thirties – your neck is just … there. Not bothering you, not causing any problems and that's fine: all we have to do is remember the sunscreen.

So for those of us who were less than careful at protecting our necks or are just wondering if neck creams are worth the extra spend the answer is both yes … and no. Definitely no if you are young; and also no if you haven't got the budget for them, because the skin on the neck isn't as wimpy as the face and can handle much richer creams, so you can confidently use your regular body moisturiser instead. Neck cream is a bit like eye cream – expensive and not usually necessary

But the answer is yes if you are of an age where crepe neck might creep up on you at any moment or if you would simply like to try a good neck cream.

Beauty tip: Easy facial exercise for jowls and neck

One of the best things you can do for your neck and jawline is to exercise it regularly. And it's so easy: no weights, treadmills or visits to the gym required.

Sit up straight in your chair and lean your head back so you can see the ceiling. Stretch your bottom lip over the top lip as far as you can until you feel the neck and jowl area tighten. Hold this position for a count of ten and then relax. Do this ten times a day and it will tighten and tone that hated crepey jowly area.

You will look like a crazed chimpanzee though, so make sure no one sees you doing it. But rest assured that even if they do, you will get the last laugh with your firm neck and jawline.

Crepe neck

Crepe neck is hated almost universally. While we have heard many a woman say that they don't mind their lines or quite like their character-forming shape, we have never heard anyone say that about crepey skin or age spots on their neck or hands. And while Susan Sarandon puts her youthful looks down to a neck procedure, this probably isn't an option for most of us.

So if you're serious about looking after your neck, make sure to cleanse it every night and give it some love with a mild AHA-based toner. Stock up on some cheaper serums and oils (they don't have to be as fancypants as the ones you use on your face) and use them all over your neck and décolletage area, rubbing them in using upward movements. Don't forget to push the skin on the jawline up towards your ears – jowls need all the help they can get to stay firm.

It's easy to spend horrendous money on neck creams. Dior, in particular, have ridiculously-priced offerings, but the good news is that creams that do well on the neck don't have to be labelled 'neck' at all: body creams are fine.

If you'd like to try a cream specifically for necks, Boots Time Delay Wrinkle Reduce Double Action Instant Tautening Gel & Anti-Ageing Cream, Mama Mio Nexercise High Protein Neck and Jawline Concentrate, Marks & Spencer Age Replenish Neck Cream and Sarah Chapman Skinesis Chest and Neck Rejuvenating Complex all get good reviews.

If you're serious about looking after your neck, make sure to cleanse it every night and give it some love with a mild AHA-based toner.

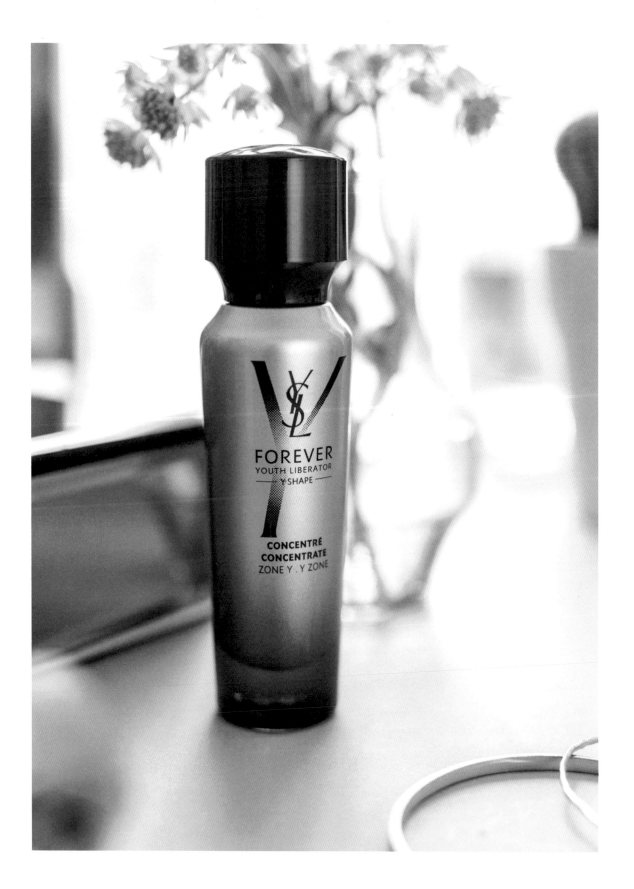

~~~~~~~~~

*Stop hunching over that laptop or iPad: keep your
shoulders back and prop your device up as high as
you can so it is close to eye level.*

~~~~~~~~~

Tech Neck

Listen, we're so used to having our insecurities preyed on in the name of the great gods of marketing with a plethora of made-up problems conspiring daily to make us self-conscious about something new. Remember the whole 'arms are the new face' thing? We can thank Michelle Obama for that as her sculpted limbs convinced every other woman on the planet that she had gross wobbly bingo wings and the cosmetic industry sold shedloads of firming creams on the back of it.

The same goes for 'your elbows are ageing you'. Cue the sale of even stronger body creams and balms designed especially for elbows. Feck's sake. And now Tech Neck is the next thing worrying everyone who has a laptop, iPhone, iPad or any of the other myriad tech devices that are in constant use.

But we have a sneaking suspicion that Tech Neck really *is* a thing. And there's no harm in taking a few preventative measures to halt its wicked onset, is there?

The problem is that every time we use our computerised devices, we look down. This is an ergonomic nightmare for the body, putting pressure on the back, the joints and especially the neck muscles.

Constantly peering down into our screens means that we put more and more pressure on our necks to hold our heads up. As the head tilts forward, the amount of weight it puts on the neck multiplies, leading not only to possible neck pain and back problems but also to the lovely added bonus of making us look saggy and baggy much earlier than we should.

Realistically, we are never going to give up our small-screen lovers so we need to improve our posture. Stop hunching over that laptop or iPad: keep your shoulders back and prop your device up as high as you can so it is close to eye level. Get gurning: facial massage and exercises do a lot to firm the jaw line – especially the deranged chimp on page 98.

Good neck creams together with regular use of SPF on the neck will help too. The neck can cope with much richer creams than the face, so try Clarins Extra-Firming Neck Anti-Wrinkle Rejuvenating Cream and Prevage Anti-Aging Neck and Decolleté Firm & Repair Cream; thick moisturisers such as Nivea Soft Refreshingly Soft Moisturising Cream will also do the job nicely. YSL Forever Youth Liberator Y-Shape Concentrate contains concentrated glycan, a sugar naturally produced by our skin that stimulates collagen renewal. As glycan pro-duction naturally declines from the age of thirty, the addition of this substance to the upper levels of skin may help.

Research is ongoing, so all of this could be blown out of the water, but perhaps glycan hold the key to unlocking, if not the fountain of youth, the path to smoother, younger-looking skin. Let's wait and see.

Apparently, Tech Neck first manifests as a line above the collar bone but before you panic and throw your iPhone away, consider this: it may be that some of us are simply more prone to developing neck lines earlier than others. A straw poll of friends who are constantly glued to their iPads revealed that the mid-forties digital marketing exec didn't have the ring above her clavicle that the twenty-something graphic designer did. Both of them do suffer from neck pain though, so it looks as if, lines aside, the real danger of Tech Neck may be the damage we are doing to our joints.

Good neck creams together with regular use of SPF on the neck will help. The neck can cope with much richer creams than the face.

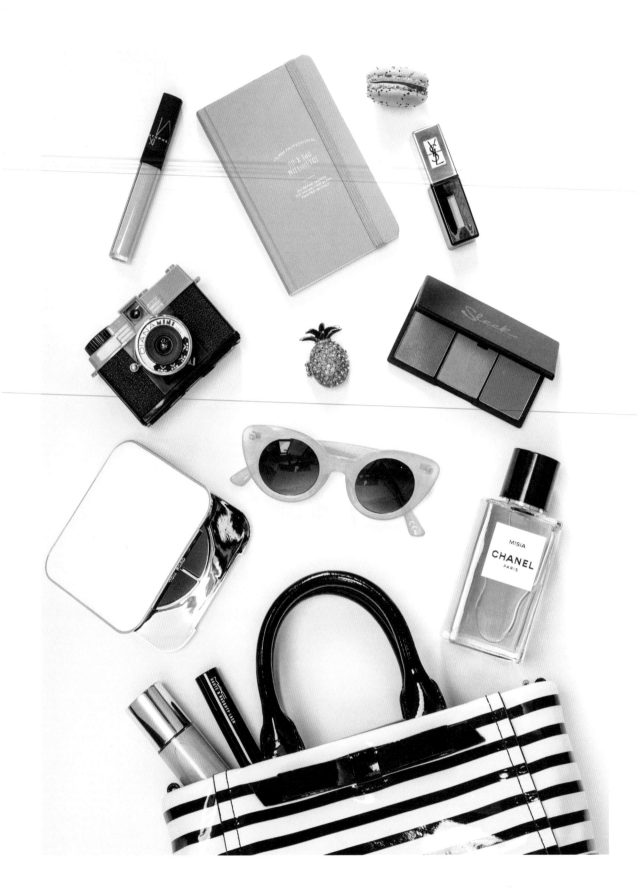

MAKE-UP

MAKE-UP • FOUNDATION • BLUSH
BRONZER AND HIGHLIGHTER • EYESHADOW • EYELINER
MASCARA • EYEBROWS • LIPSTICK

CHAPTER 10

· MAKE-UP ·

rish women have boundless enthusiasm for make-up. We spend more on it and wear more of it than our European counterparts, and our lust for new shades and formulations is never sated. It's time to take a moment to think about the positives of that relationship. We can use make-up to express ourselves, to convey whatever mood we're in on a given day, and to enhance our best features to make them even better. Sometimes the shadows underneath our eyes can make us forget that they're actually big, or wonderfully angled, or adorned with incredible eyelashes. We don't need make-up, and it can't necessarily give us features we don't have, but it helps us to make the very most of what we do have. It's a riot of colour, texture and fragrance. Just being around it can make you feel good.

Make-up has transformative power, and that's meaningful. You can use a lot of it to create a look, or a little. We want you to feel good in your make-up every day. Regardless of your age, gender and any other factor, make-up can make your day a little brighter and a little easier to get through. On an off day, it can make you feel more like yourself. On a good day, it can give you a confidence boost that makes you feel able for anything. There's something magical about its power, and even after years of lipsticks, swaths of eyeshadow and approximately eighty-six litres of emergency concealer, we're still completely entranced by make-up.

Laura had her first experience of serious make-up embarrassingly late. During Leaving Cert year, the artiest girl in the class sauntered in one morning with sparkly emerald eyeshadow, and a love affair was born (with make-up, not the arty girl. This isn't that kind of story.). 'Where did you get that green stuff?' Laura asked her in a whisper. 'It's Mac, of course,' the arty girl replied with mysterious confidence. Laura had somehow managed to reach eighteen in Ireland without knowing about Mac – quite a feat, considering that Brown Thomas's Mac counter in Dublin is second in sales only to Bloomingdale's in New York. That green eyeshadow mesmerised her enough to send her, terrified and clueless, into Brown Thomas the next day. She left with a sparkling amber eyeshadow of her very own, and an altered world view.

Make-up is just a little thing, a frippery. Yet it's little things that enrich you and make you feel good. In this respect, make-up punches well above its weight. If one budget foundation can help us muster the confidence to get through an interview or one slick of lip gloss can brighten a bad day, then make-up is far more powerful than we give it credit for.

So that's what we're doing in this section. Make-up is not something to be frightened of, or to feel bad about. You're its master, not the other way round, and there really aren't any solid rules. Make-up is about freedom. It's your face – do whatever makes you happy.

The basic kit: Make-up

Over the course of her lifetime, every woman will accrue a make-up collection. For some, it will consist of a few well-loved eyeliners and some lip balm. For others, it will be a vast array of complex products that require some expertise to apply. What you want in your collection is up to you, but if you're starting from scratch, there are some basics that every kit can use.

Not everyone wears foundation, but if you do, be aware that you'll probably need to have two. Depending on your skin tone, you'll always be one or more shades deeper in summer than in winter. Even if you're diligent with SPF, mild everyday sun exposure will darken your skin over the summer months, so it's best to have two foundations – a lighter shade for summer and a deeper shade for winter. The formulation you choose will depend on your skin type and the amount of coverage you want.

A brow product helps to define eyebrows and bring structure to the face, while an eyeshadow quad containing four neutral shades works for any situation, day or night. You can branch out and buy more eyeshadows whenever you want, but a starter collection doesn't need any more than four. A good mascara does wonders for tired eyes, and blush puts balance back into a face after foundation has evened out skin tone. Add a couple of lipsticks – a bold colour and an understated nude – to complete any make-up collection.

The basic kit: Tools

The availability of quality brushes at any price range is better than it's ever been – we're literally spoilt for choice. But if you find the whole brush thing a bit baffling, then having so much choice and so many questions to answer doesn't necessarily help.

Brushes are great, but only when they actually enhance the make-up application. If fingers will do the job, then use those instead. So if you're looking to build a little wardrobe of very reliable basic make-up brushes, then go for the essentials – brushes which do a job that fingers can't.

A basic set of brushes should include a great angled brush for gel liner (synthetic bristles create the smoothest finish) and a natural-fibre angled brush for brow powders and gels. A good fluffy blush brush can be used for powder blush, bronzer and foundation. And a fluffy eyeshadow brush is essential for good eye make-up – nothing else will produce that smooth, blended finish that we all covet.

Make sure to experiment. Natural-fibre fluffy brushes (such as blush brushes) can be fantastic for buffing on foundation. Laura discovered this when studying make-up artistry after years of being told that this was an absolute no-no. If you like the effect produced, keep doing whatever you're doing.

If you're investing in your first set of good brushes, opt for high-quality affordable

Brushes are great, but only when they will actually enhance the make-up application. If fingers will do the job, then use those instead

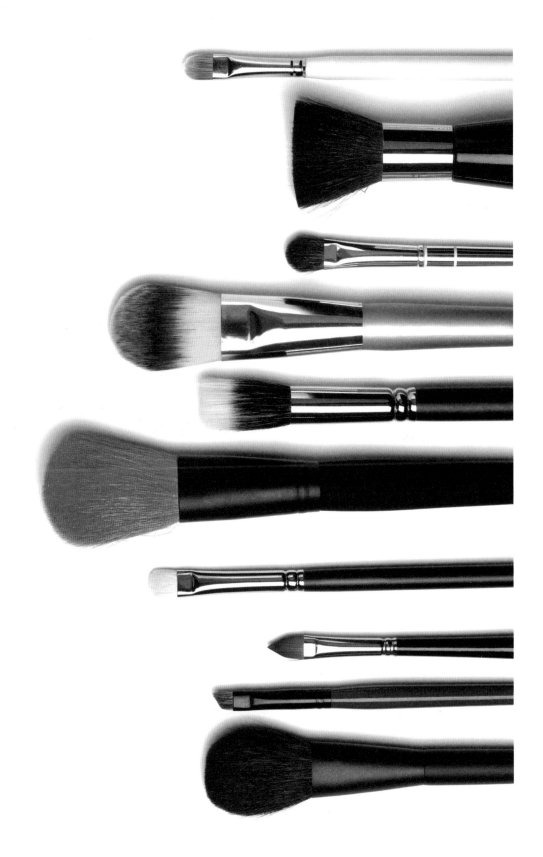

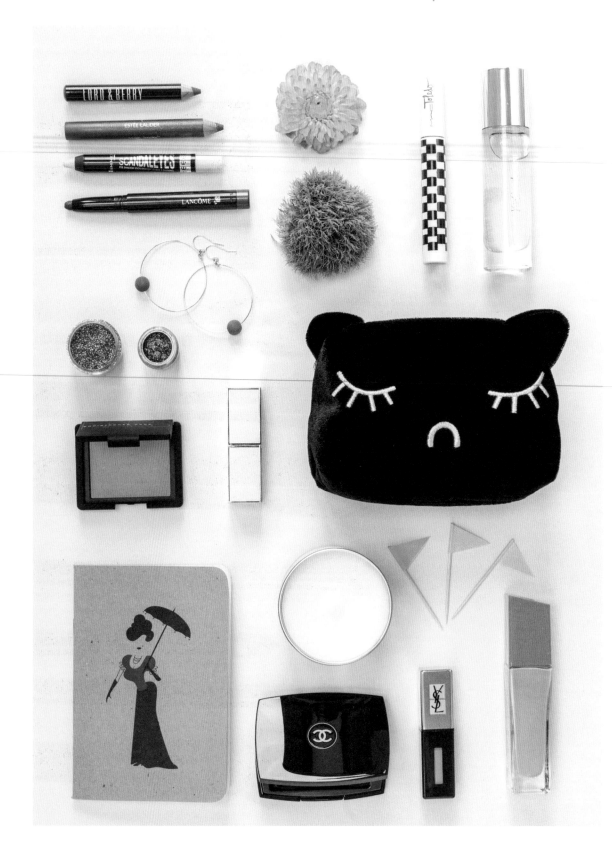

Beauty decoded: Blend

Blend: Using a fluffy brush to blur away any harsh edges or streaks in the product.

Beauty tutorial: How to blend

Remember with all brushes that where you hold them is important. For blending eyeshadow, hold the brush at the very back of the handle – this prevents you from putting pressure on the tip and ensures lightness of touch and a properly buffed finish. Be patient with blending. It's a matter of sticking with it until a globby mess has transformed into a smoky wonder. Keep at it and it will happen – you can correct any errors with a touch of concealer. Just remember to blend, blend and blend until you see the smooth results you were hoping for.

brands like Real Techniques and Crown. Crown have a great contour brush that works brilliantly for powder blush and bronzer, but Laura loves to use it for foundation. And Real Techniques' brilliantly unassuming Setting Brush is one of our favourite brushes because it's such a great multitasker. It buffs concealer and foundation seamlessly and can be used to set hard to reach places with powder. In a fix, it will even blend eyeshadow.

Mac's 224 Tapered Blending Brush is a thing of beauty. Blending powder eyeshadow to create that smoky effect is something only a brush can do, so if you like to wear blended eye make-up every day, this is entirely worth the investment.

Concealing can be a tricky business using just your fingers. For the fiddly work and pinpoint concealing of little blemishes, a small fluffy brush is what we prefer. Try the Real Techniques Shading Brush, which we love. Its synthetic fibres don't absorb too much product and the tiny brush-head makes concealing in fiddly areas, like under brows or the sides of the nose, a breeze. And yes, while it's technically for eyeshadow, we like making our brushes multitask. That's why we like Real Techniques – the brushes are affordable, excellent quality and good multitaskers.

Once you feel ready to graduate onto some more skill-specific brushes, you might like to invest in a flat contour brush like the 301 from the Real Techniques Bold Metals range or the Mac 163 Flat Contour Brush. These are brilliant for cream products, like blush and contour, and can also be used for foundation if you're feeling experimental.

Concealing can be a tricky business using just your fingers. For the fiddly work and pinpoint concealing of little blemishes, a small fluffy brush is what we prefer.

CHAPTER 11

· FOUNDATION ·

Foundation is the product that women tell us stresses them out most, and for good reason. No matter how beautifully applied a face of make-up may be, if your foundation is the wrong colour or formulation, then your make-up will look weird and shabby, as though you started applying fake tan from the head down but lost interest around your chin.

Foundation is about creating an illusion. If you have perfect skin, you don't need to wear any. Though we rely on foundation a bit too much for coverage here in Ireland, it really is intended as a product to even skin tone and not as a cover-all for disguising blemishes or blotting out pigmentation.

Since foundation is all about creating an effect on the skin, its focus is more on function than skincare. Ingredients are tailored to create the right texture on the surface, rather than to manipulate what's happening beneath it – and that's no bad thing.

A good skincare routine will keep your skin happy, so that you can wear less make-up (if you want to) and experience the supreme satisfaction of applying a little foundation and watching it sit perfectly on the skin. Covering skin texture is not foundation's job – it's there to even out skin tone so don't cake it on.

It's not essential to wear foundation, but if you're going to wear it, then it has to match your skin perfectly. Achieving this is less scary than it seems, though we've all had mismatch horror stories.

Foundation shopping can be every bit as traumatic as attempting to buy jeans right after Christmas when you've eaten your own body weight in stuffing. If you're feeling a bit vulnerable, then put off the search for a new foundation until you're robust enough to navigate the obstacle course of department store beauty counters. Unless you're feeling confident, the world of perfume clouds, overly friendly counter assistants and endless foundation shades and choices will have you cowering in a corner and whimpering within a few minutes.

There's absolutely nothing wrong with asking for a sample of any foundation that you're interested in buying, so don't feel uncomfortable about it. Traditionally, beauty brands in Ireland aren't very forthcoming with samples, but certain outlets and brands are great for giving samples.

Beauty tip: Counter etiquette

In most cases, we have found that if you are nice to make-up counter assistants, then they're nice back. For every horror story we hear about bad customer experiences, we have plenty of feedback from the other side of the counter too. Shops are fed up with people coming along and taking up tons of their time getting swatched and matched before taking a note of the shades that suit them and going home to buy them online. Customers can be as rude as the most tangoed counter assistant, so make sure you're nice as pie and all should go smoothly. If it doesn't, just put it down to experience and don't worry about it.

Neither of us have ever had a bad experience at a make-up counter and we wondered why, considering the terrible tales we'd heard from other women. So in a daring experiment, Laura went undercover to find out for once and for all what the hell was happening in some of our department stores. Yes, we will stop at nothing in our quest to seek out the truth. In she went to a posh department store, dressed in a scruffy tracksuit, with slightly scuzzy hair and no make-up, and approached a counter with some basic questions about foundation.

After being treated quite dismissively – because apparently a cruddy tracksuit means that you know jack-all about make-up – she left with an orange face, despite the fact that she knew her correct shade-match before going in.

The less you know about make-up, the more willing a counter assistant should be to take the time to help and to be friendly. Many are, but it doesn't hurt at the very least to do your research before you head into the shops so you can tell if you're being steered wrong. It often helps to bring an empty sample bottle with you, so there's no excuse not to give you a sample.

And perhaps wash your tracksuit while you're at it.

In most cases, we have found that if you are nice to make-up counter assistants, then they're nice back.

Choosing your foundation

There are loads of really talented make-up artists on beauty counters around Ireland. There are also lots of duds. Often, make-up artists at department store counters are simply reproducing the make-up they feel works most for themselves on their customers, and that's pretty much never a recipe for success. It's important to be educated as a consumer and to be able to rely on your own knowledge when buying a new foundation. Trusted advice is always helpful, but self-reliance will never steer you wrong.

There are two major factors to consider when buying foundation: formulation and shade. Get either wrong, and you're on a fast track to orange porridge face. The formulation needs to suit your skin type; for example, a moisturising foundation will nestle snugly onto dry skin but will slip right off an oily skin and may well just take your eye make-up with it on its travels. No one wants to look as though they've just worn a full face of make-up to a sauna, so proceed carefully.

For example, Laura loves the formulation of Mac Studio Sculpt Foundation, and it looks great on her for a short time. Since it has a moist formulation, it slides off as the natural oiliness of her skin starts to come through from underneath. By the end of the day, there's nothing but shine left, and some blotches of foundation in her face's drier areas. Definitely not a good look. She can lust after it all she likes, but it just isn't going to look as good on her as it does on someone else.

Take that same foundation and put it on Aisling's dry skin, and you have a match made in heaven – the moistness marries with her drier skin to produce a dewy effect that looks fresh and glowy all day. Wanting to love a foundation that's just plain wrong for your skin type is a bit like admiring a dress on someone else when you know you just won't suit your figure. What you're really envying in that situation is the fact that someone looks great, and you always look great when you tailor what you're wearing to your shape and colouring. Tailor your foundation to your skin tone and type, and you're away. You'll have people complimenting your skin in no time and you can be all casual about it, which is always fun.

Counter assistants have to wear a lot of make-up, and it's designed to look good under department store lighting. Out in the real world, in daylight, it can look a bit drag-like so it's just not necessarily suited to grocery shopping in Aldi on a Wednesday afternoon. So although you should always take the advice of beauty counter assistants into account, your safest bet is to be able to shade-match yourself.

It's challenging to shade-match other people because it involves understanding a variety of skin tones and the undertones which compose them. But you only need to shade-match one person – yourself. Developing the skill to do this properly will eliminate half the stress of shopping for foundation.

Here's how to do it.

- Much as it may fill you with terror, it is best

to go foundation shopping with a bare face – that way you're guaranteed to find the right match.

- Before you go, think about the brands you're interested in and the formulation you think will suit you best.

- To make sure you have enough time to do this at your leisure, we suggest you go into department stores in the morning. If you head in on a weekday morning before 11:00 am, you'll be able to take your time and have a good browse without dealing with crowds of make-up-obsessed teenagers sampling products in a horrifyingly unhygienic manner.

- Pick out the three shades that you think are probably most likely to match – not the colour you wish you were, but the colour that you think you actually are. If you want something to match your skin when you are wearing fake tan, wear the tan on your shopping trip to ensure a perfect match.

- Swatch your three potential shades vertically on your jawline. The darker your skin tone, the more likely that your skin will have areas of different shades. If you have a darker skin tone, you may need two foundation shades to achieve a realistic effect, a slightly lighter shade in the centre of your face and a deeper one for the outer edges. Swatch along the jaw down onto the neck and onto the forehead to assess which shades your skin needs.

- If you're just going with a jawline swatch, then the shade that disappears into your skin is the right shade for you. Ideally, you should head into the nearest daylight to find out for sure. If none of the three you've chosen disappear, then go back to the counter, take the next three that look like good candidates to you, and try again. Keep going until one swatch disappears into your skin – that's the one for you. You've found it. Job done. Go and have a scone, because you've found the right foundation without any crisis at all.

Beauty decoded: Ingredients in foundation

As well as finding the perfect shade you may also need additional qualities from a foundation. Let's demystify what makes up a foundation.

Titanium dioxide is used for pigment in foundations, but it also acts as a physical sunblock. It's the light of a camera flash bouncing off this ingredient that causes Ghost Face in photos (page 70), so opt for an SPF-free formulation if there will be a photographer anywhere near you. SPF 15 or under will probably be safe for photographing, but if you're at all nervous of flashback, opt for an SPF-free formulation. For the perfect photo-ready foundation, we recommend Revlon PhotoReady Makeup, as well as Make Up For Ever HD Loose Setting Powder and Laura Mercier Loose Setting Powder.

Mica, frequently used in HD foundations, creates that nice pearlescent, light-reflective finish that everyone loves in more radiant foundations, but as it's a mineral, you'll often find it in classic powder formulations too, like bareMinerals Original Foundation and Lily Lolo Mineral Foundation SPF 15.

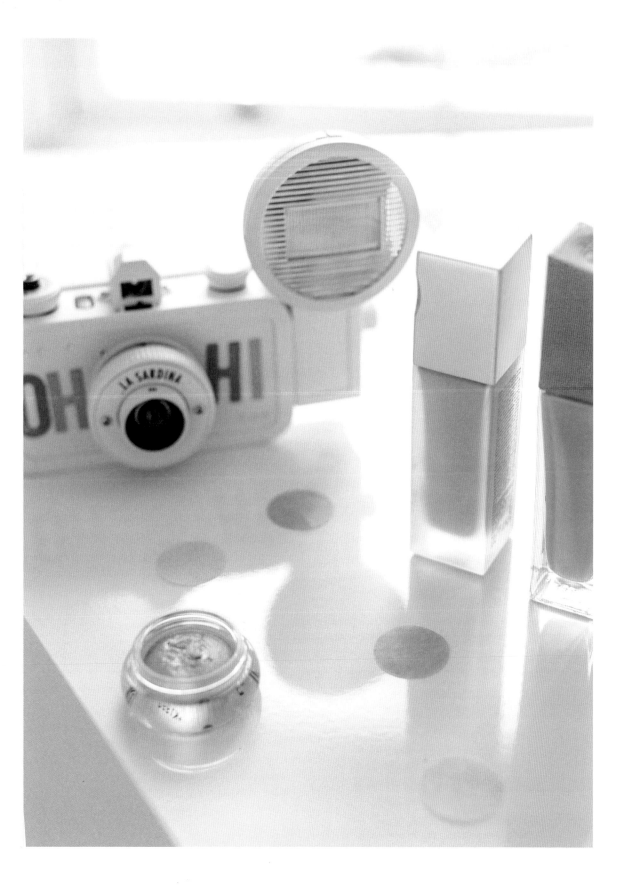

Silicones are everywhere – you'll find them in hair products as well as in primers and foundations. They are generally used to give products a bit of slip on the skin and to act as a filler, to create that smoothing layer between skin and foundation, which ensures that products sit nicely on the skin. This is because silicone molecules are too large to be absorbed into the skin. Silicone ingredients are generally listed as dimethicone, but anything ending in -cone or -zane is a silicone.

It's a rare liquid foundation that is silicone-free because they keep the foundation looking fresh, make it easy to apply and stop it from drying out and looking flaky. While some people don't like silicones, our policy is to make the most of what's available. If your skin seems to get on well with them, use them.

Beauty decoded: Foundation undertone

The 'pink or yellow' undertone conundrum has been confusing women since the dawn of foundation. Basically, everyone's skin has an undertone and to make your foundation look natural, you have to make sure you're wearing the right tone for you. Pink is also referred to as 'cool' and yellow as 'warm'.

The only exception to this rule is Mac, who very frustratingly operate a completely opposite system, but it's less confusing than it sounds and we'll cover that in a bit.

Bobbi Brown famously declared that 99% of women, with the exception of the super-pale, have yellow undertones to their skin, so Bobbi Brown only make yellow-toned foundation. It makes sense: most people around the world do indeed have yellow undertone. The problem is that many of the small global percentage of pink-undertoned people live right here in Ireland, and many foundations with yellow undertones won't do a thing for us.

A yellow undertone is generally found on people with darker-toned skin – Asian and Hispanic people, for example, have that lovely golden hue, so their undertone is obviously more yellow than pink.

People with darker skin can also have a red undertone, so finding a foundation match can sometimes be a bit more complicated, as tones in darker skin often show more variation than in lighter skin. Just remember, your ideal foundation will match your undertone.

A pink undertone is found on people with sun-sensitive, paler skin. So if you are positively bacon-like after ten minutes in the sun, odds are your undertone is pink. Equally, if your skin tans in the sun and doesn't tend to burn, then you have a yellow undertone.

Of course, that's a simplification, because some people are neutral, but thankfully there is a glut of foundations on the market now that contain both pink and yellow undertones, so there will always be something out there to match you.

For a quick and easy way to find out which you are, so you don't waste money on the wrong products trying to find the right ones, look at the colour of the veins in your wrist. As a general rule, if they're blue, then you are pink-toned. If they're green, then you are yellow-toned, because the tone of your skin alters the colour of the veins.

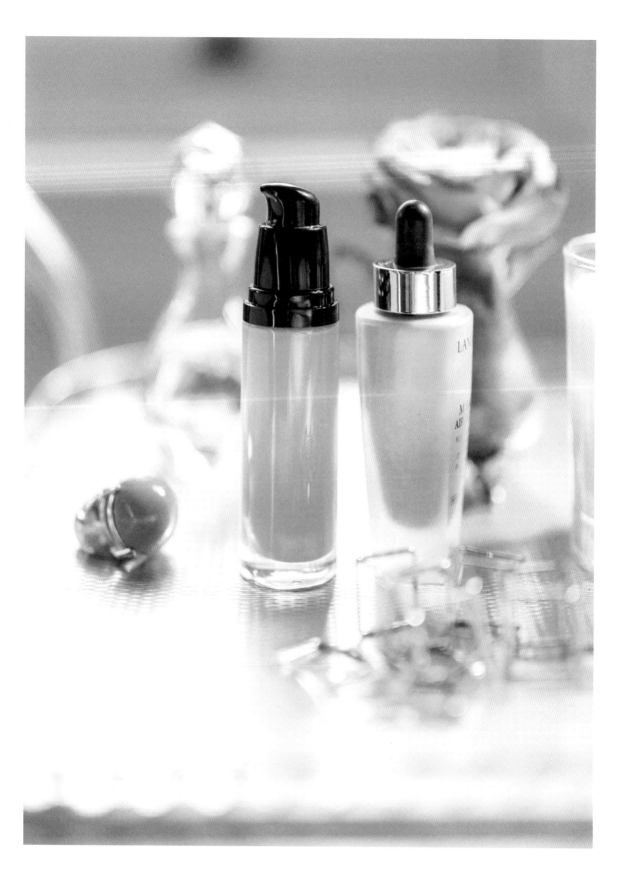

If you're still uncertain, go to a beauty counter with a make-up-free face and apply some pink-toned foundation (it'll look pinkish in the bottle) to one side of your jawline, following the same method you'd use for foundation matching (page 113), and a yellow-toned foundation (it will look yellower in the bottle) on the other. The guide for finding the right foundation is exactly the same as standard foundation matching – the one that disappears is the right one for you.

YSL Le Teint Touche Éclat Foundation offers a wide range of foundation shades in pink, yellow and neutral undertones. The BD (Beige Doré) shades are for those with yellow undertones, the BR (Beige Rose) shades are for pink undertones and the B shades (Beige) are more neutral. While Bobbi Brown foundations all have a yellow undertone, their palest shade – Alabaster, which is only available in some of the foundation formulas – is for pinker skins.

As we mentioned, Mac's system is different, but it's nothing to be scared of. It follows the same principle, but they switch things around. They have two foundation groups – NW and NC. NW tones mean 'neutral warm', which are actually for cooler, pink undertones. NC or 'neutral cool' is for warmer, yellower skin tones. It's all a bit confusing. If you're overwhelmed, stick to the swatch test. If it disappears into your skin, you've found the right one.

Cheaper foundations can be pink and yellow too – Maybelline and L'Oréal both distinguish between tones. However, if the brand you've chosen doesn't distinguish between pink and yellow undertones, don't worry. A lot of brands don't tell you if they base their shades on cool (pink) or warm (yellow) undertones. Just do the jawline test and pick the foundation that blends in best with your skin. Higher-end foundation tends to distinguish more often between pink and yellow, perhaps because these brands tend to offer a lot more choice in shades.

There's no need to get too bogged down in undertones. They're good to keep in mind as a guideline when choosing shades to test on your skin in your search for the right one, but you can find the right shade even without knowing anything about undertones. Just follow our technique for a perfect colour match, and the undertone will take care of itself.

If the brand you've chosen doesn't distinguish between pink and yellow undertones, don't worry. Just do the jawline test and pick the foundation that blends in best with your skin.

Primer

Primer is a nice addition to your make-up bag for special occasions, but it's not an essential everyday product. If you're going to be photographed and your make-up needs to last, primer can help. If your skin is particularly oily or the climate is particularly hot, a mattifying primer can give your foundation some grip and help keep it in place. An illuminating primer can give glow to duller, drier skin to help make-up sit better.

Though Laura Mercier Foundation Primer in Radiance is a touch too slick for people with very oily skin, it gives an incomparable glow to skin even before you apply foundation. Eliminating the need for a separate liquid highlighter, this looks fantastic under make-up and gives an all-over glow with the extra benefit of blurring the complexion just a little. If your skin is dry, this helps to prevent that nasty sitting effect that foundation can develop after several hours' wear. Hourglass Veil has a velvet texture and the added benefit of SPF 15, which is generally too low to cause Ghost Face in photos, making this an all-round great day foundation or evening primer.

Bourjois Happy Light Matte Serum Primer is an affordable wonder. Feather-light but hard-working, it creates an invisible matte veil that keeps skin shine-free. If you're oilier around the centre of the face, just wear this around the t-zone area to stay matte and to minimise touch-ups, although no matter what make-up you use, at least one touch-up per day will probably be needed to keep everything looking fresh. It also comes in a more luminous version for drier skins.

Benefit The Porefessional is one of the best primers for evening skin texture. Dabbed just around the nose and forehead, it minimises shine and blurs away pores. If silicone textures don't bother you and you don't mind the poly-filla effect from time to time, the Porefessional will cheat good skin for you. On a budget, Catrice Prime and Fine Smoothing Refiner do a similar job.

Smashbox Photo Finish Foundation Primer is a bestseller for a reason and comes in several different versions, all of which glide onto skin for a veil of sheer loveliness that works for all skin types. For a more affordable version of this classic with less glow, try L'Oréal Infallible Mattifying Primer. For oilier skins, Bioderma Sébium Pore Refiner Corrective Concentrate is a good pre-foundation option for anyone concerned about breakthrough shine or oversized pores.

Foundation brushes

There's no need to use a foundation brush if you prefer to use your fingers because they give more control than a brush, and the pressure with which you tap the product into the skin can create different effects. Famed make-up artist Mary Greenwell always applies foundation to models with her hands – her method can look hilariously slap-dab, with hands flying all over the place and lots of face grabbing, but when she's finished, the effect is always flawless and highly skilled. So don't feel that you 'have' to use a foundation brush – just go with whatever suits you.

Aisling never uses a foundation brush and when Laura does use a brush for foundation (most of the time she applies foundations with her fingers), she refuses to use a standard old-fashioned flat foundation brush.

In fact, she hates them with a passion. The product sits on them, they streak and they never produce a nice, buffed finish. Don't think for an instant that you can't use a brush for any purpose other than the one written on the side. Natural-fibre fluffy brushes, such as blush brushes, can be fantastic for buffing on foundation, even though some people are horrified by the idea of it. Experiment with your brushes and nuts to the rules. If you like the effect a brush creates, even if you're using it unconventionally, then keep doing whatever you're doing because it works.

Crown's Contour Brush works beautifully for its stated purpose, powder blush and bronzer, but it also works brilliantly for applying liquid foundation in little flicky motions. The Buffing Brush from Real Techniques is very reasonably priced and it buffs foundation or cream cheek products into the skin for a perfect airbrushed finish that looks like flawless skin.

Beauty decoded: Buff

Buff: A vigorous swirling motion using a fluffy brush, by which you rub foundation seamlessly into the skin.

Natural-fibre, fluffy brushes, such as blush brushes, can be fantastic for buffing on foundation.

Powder

Powder is one of those enduring products throughout the history of make-up, the sort of product that has a bad reputation because your granny used too much of it. Formulations and textures are thankfully a lot silkier and less antiquated than they used to be, and powder brush isn't just for oily skin. Applied with a fluffy powder brush and pressed into the skin, it will set and mattify foundation without displacing it. Avoid dragging the brush across the skin – that will move and streak foundation.

Powder foundations are brilliant for setting dewy make-up and adding an extra layer of coverage. Mac Studio Fix Powder Plus Foundation is finely milled to keep it from looking clogged and unnatural on the skin, and leaves skin looking perfectly even, but not dry. Giorgio Armani Luminous Silk Powder mimics the famous Armani foundation it takes its name from and is consequently divine.

Rimmel Stay Matte Pressed Powder is a more affordable option that still goes the distance. The shade range is less extensive than those from Mac or Giorgio Armani, but it comes in a transparent option to suit all skin tones. Chanel Les Beiges Healthy Glow Sheer Powder is a delicious, finely-milled powder which will add a touch of coverage while it luminously mattifies, while NYC Smooth Skin Pressed Face Powder is a nice affordable option.

If you prefer loose powders, Laura Mercier Loose Setting Powder is a classically reliable choice, and Clinique Blended Face Powder is perfect for drier and more mature skins.

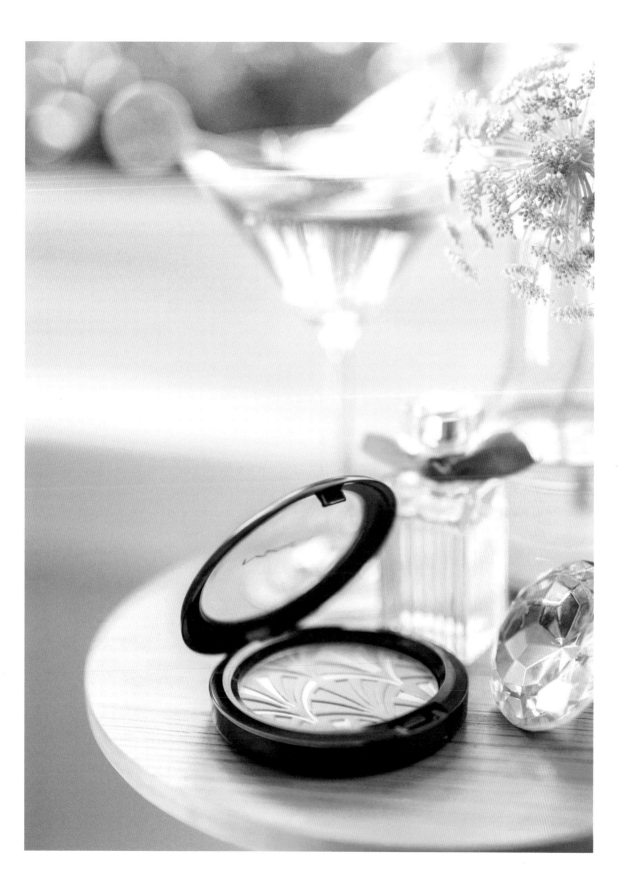

Beauty tip: Setting spray

If powder isn't your bag, then a modern setting spray is a quick and easy option that you can reapply as often as you like. Mac Prep+Prime Fix+ and Urban Decay All Nighter Makeup Setting Spray are great. Hold the bottle a few inches from you face and spritz. As it dries, it sets your make-up. It can also be used to liven up drab, day-old make-up.

Beauty tip: Avoiding the dreaded Foundation Moustache

Aisling has a thing about facial hair. Like many grandmothers, hers had an impressive face of fuzz that had to be razed into oblivion when it got out of control, and Aisling is terrified of inheriting this beard. Just like Granny, she has thick, dark hair, pale skin and the odd whisker that seems to suddenly spring forth fully grown.

Forget Movember being just for the men – we know plenty of women who could join in and grow a full-on tache. Without vigorous pruning, many of us could challenge Tom Selleck in a tache-growing competition. Many of us wax, tweeze, laser, thread and even burn the faces off ourselves with depilatory cream, all in the pursuit of a smooth upper lip and chin. Some women employ methods that are barbaric, to say the least. Most hair-removal techniques are at best temporary (there's no such thing as permanent hair removal, despite what the laser clinics tell you) and most of them hurt like hell.

Even if you have fair or red hair, you probably identify with at least some of this. And even though your facial hair might be fine and downy and not immediately visible, putting on foundation often throws any hair on your face into relief, thickens it and instantly creates a Foundation Moustache. This is one of nature's cruellest tricks. At least dark-haired women know all about their moustaches and have had the opportunity to whip them away.

If you've noticed this happening and aren't happy about it, then there are lots of things you can do to make it all less visible.

Application is crucial. If your normal method of applying foundation is to just rub it in with your fingers or swipe it on with a brush, then you're probably applying foundation from side to side as well as up and down. This means hairs are coated fully from every angle and will stand out proudly in a thick and luscious manner. Instead, use a stippling brush and lightly pat foundation in downward strokes. This will make hair lie flat and will only cover one surface.

Many people find that liquid foundation is too thick and sticky and clings to hair, so mineral foundation is a really good choice for the upper-lip area. You can still use your liquid foundation on the rest of your face and just use mineral make-up on your upper lip or sideburns. Buff in a minimal amount with a large fluffy brush, and make sure you brush downwards to flatten the hairs.

Do not even think of applying powder on top of foundation to this area. Powder will bulk up the hairs even more.

Most hair-removal techniques are at best temporary (there's no such thing as permanent hair removal, despite what the laser clinics tell you) and most of them hurt like hell.

The best foundation for each skin type

BALANCED SKIN

What a lot of people in the beauty industry call 'normal skin', we've decided to refer to in this section as 'balanced'. The majority of us don't have balanced skin, so imbalance is pretty normal. By 'balanced' skin, we really just mean skin that behaves itself – not problematically oily or dry, and comfortable to live in. No one is perfect, so the occasional skin misbehaviour or breakout is completely normal.

If you're one of those lucky people who doesn't have to deal with a recurring issue like dryness or oiliness, you're balanced – and the envy of everyone.

BEST MEDIUM COVERAGE

Medium-coverage foundation is an odd beast. It's something that you can build up for nearly full-coverage if you want to, but can also sheer down if it suits your mood. It offers far more coverage than something like a tinted moisturiser, but without the sometimes oppressively thick consistency of a full-coverage base.

Medium-coverage bases are the ones we keep for nights out, special occasions (particularly if there will be photos) and bad skin days. If you wake up and all your fears have come to pass – you have a weird rash thing or your skin looks completely dull and blotchy, as though you've been dredged from a river – then reach for the medium-coverage foundation.

Nars Sheer Glow Foundation is a trusted classic. You can build this up for impressive coverage or just buff a little bit into the skin to dispel the worst of the horror and restore the impression of some sort of order to your face.

If you want medium coverage without any heaviness, Dior Airflash Spray Foundation is pleasantly strange. A lightweight spray, you can spray it directly onto the face (protect your hair at all costs as it gets all over the place) or spray it onto the back of your hand and apply it with a brush for a slightly more built-up finish. Professional make-up artists often provide an airbrush foundation service for special occasions like weddings – it's the foundation version of a spray tan. Estée Lauder gives a mean airbrush service at their counters.

Old-fashioned stick foundations get a lot of bad press, mostly because the formulation of them used to be downright disgusting. These days, they're more intelligent and Bobbi Brown Skin Foundation Stick is one of the very best. Apply directly to prepped skin and buff out with fingers or a brush. This is one of the few Bobbi Brown foundations which is still available in Alabaster, the brand's super-pale shade, as well as a veritable rainbow of other shades. NYX Mineral Stick Foundation is another good stick foundation, which, unlike the Bobbi Brown version, has a matte finish.

BEST LIGHT COVERAGE

'Light coverage' isn't generally uttered with any form of admiration in Ireland. We tend to like our foundations to be more pound cake than meringue. But that doesn't mean there's no market for lighter coverage, just that we don't tend to grace light-coverage products with the honourable title of 'foundation'.

Over the years, products offering less coverage have morphed into new forms and go by new names. Tinted moisturisers, BB creams and their ilk are all light-coverage bases for good skin days, summer holidays and any other time you feel like wearing them. Do remember though that these products are essentially pigment mixed with emollients and other skincare ingredients, so you could actually make your own in a jiffy by adding a touch of your favourite foundation to some of your favourite moisturiser. Clarins Radiance-Plus Golden Glow Booster is a brilliant product to mix with your moisturiser.

Origins A Perfect World SPF 15 BB Age Defence Tinted Moisturiser with White Tea is a nice light everyday product. It comes in a decent shade range of six colours and is very pleasantly moisturising. YSL Le Teint Touche Éclat Foundation was ten years in the making, which may explain why we find it perfection. Suitable for all skin types (though you may need a touch of powder if you're on the oily side), a little bit will create a radiant glow, and you can build it almost to medium coverage if you want to. It's certainly a foundation that defies definition, though it's on the lighter side of the spectrum.

Rimmel Match Perfection Foundation is a dead ringer for YSL's famed Le Teint Touche Éclat Foundation, but at a far more affordable price. Candlelit skin in a bottle is an understatement. This works for all skin types, but oilier skin will need to be set with a powder.

Over the years, products offering less coverage have morphed into new forms and go by new names. Tinted moisturisers, BB creams and their ilk are all light-coverage bases for good skin days, summer holidays and any other time you feel like wearing them.

OILY SKIN

Though oily skin is the plague of its owner, you're really quite lucky to have it. And yes, we know that's what your granny used to say while she pinched your cheeks with an agonising power you never thought such feeble little hands could muster, but she wasn't wrong.

At the risk of sounding a bit trite, when your skin is being oily, it's not being dry, and dry skin can be hard to apply make-up over. If your oily skin is acne-prone, then that's another story. A few blemishes are easy as pie to cover up, but lots of difference in texture is more difficult. Start an appropriate skincare routine for your skin type and you will ensure the best possible canvas for your make-up.

If your skincare routine really works for your skin and it's well-behaved in all aspects, except its bag-of-chips tendency to seep through whatever you put on it, then that's just your skin type and you've got to work with it.

Oil-absorbing ingredients are the oily person's best friend. Matte textures and silica will absorb excess sebum and help your base to stay in place all day, as will an oil-free matte primer. A certain amount of acceptance of reality is required though. Touch-ups will be needed, because your skin is a live organ, constantly working.

Women with oily skin have never had it better when it comes to foundations. The new formulas are light, often feel weightless on the skin and although they are incredibly fluid, still provide very good coverage and can last all day without re-application. Our oily-skinned testers have been on a mission to find the best on the market. Our criteria: foundations that keep oiliness in check for as long as possible and leave skin feeling comfortable while looking natural.

BEST MEDIUM COVERAGE

If your skin is oily, acne-prone and blemished, you will love Laura Mercier Smooth Finish Flawless Fluide Foundation. It is very matte and puts up a fight against dreaded shine. It blends very easily, and the choice of more than twenty shades means there is sure to be one to suit your skin colour. The coverage lasts all day without any need for powder. Just make sure to give it a good shake before each use as some of the ingredients can settle.

In a blind testing, we challenge anyone to detect that Rimmel Stay Matte Liquid Mousse Foundation costs less than expensive foundations as it performs just as well as many of its higher-priced counterparts. Only a tiny amount is needed to cover a full face. It masks blemishes without looking heavy and lasts all day with a dab of blotting paper or powder. Catrice All Matt Plus Shine Control Make Up is another good budget buy.

Clarins Ever Matte Foundation is universally loved by oily-skinned women because it suits almost everyone, regardless of age. It provides all-day coverage with a comfortable non-shine finish that does not look overly matte. Make sure to exfoliate well to stop the formula from clinging to any flaky or dry patches.

Water-based foundations are ideal for oily skin as they do not weigh it down or add additional shine. Although Nars All Day Luminous Weightless Foundation has 'luminous' in its title, do not worry: it will not add shimmer. Instead, this means that the coverage is not a flat matte and you will find that although the formulation is extremely liquid, it only takes a scant half-pump to cover your whole face and to cancel out any redness and blemishes.

For those with truly oily skin, a powder foundation is often a good option. It doesn't smother the skin with heavy product, but it does offer the crucial oil absorbency that you need. Urban Decay Naked Skin Ultra Definition Powder Foundation is a full-coverage powder foundation. It can be used beautifully over any foundation to mattify and add a bit of extra coverage; alone or over a mattifying primer, this finely-milled lovely smooths and give coverage while absorbing excess oil.

Mac make fantastic foundations for oily skin. Their foundations are generally targeted at a younger market in which oiliness is a key skin concern. Mac Studio Fix Fluid Foundation is an absolute classic. So devoted are the pale-skinned among us to it that Mac have brought out two shades – NW10 and NW13 – specifically for pale skin tones. This foundation sits beautifully on the skin and offers more of a demi-matte finish than a basic matte. It still manages to be light-reflective and lovely, despite its staying power.

Illamasqua is still available in Ireland, but only online from Debenhams or the brand's website. Its Skin Base is a special foundation. There's just something different about it, and since it is a brand for make-up artists, like Mac, the shade range is fantastic, catering for every possible skin colour and undertone. A tiny bit will work wonders.

YSL Fusion Ink Foundation is another semi-matte offering. It's matte enough to offer oil absorption and provide grip, but it doesn't sit lazily in the pores or look dull. This is a particularly nice option for more mature but oily skin. This foundation seems so thin that you may think it cannot make any difference, but you would be wrong as oily and combination skin will be mattified, the look of pores will be diminished and skin tone evened. For even longer shine control if your skin is very oily, try Lancôme Teint Idole Ultra 24H Foundation.

Max Factor Face Finity All Day Flawless 3 in 1 Foundation is a pharmacy option that rivals department store foundations in its coverage and lasting power. Best for oilier or balanced skins, this demi-matte foundation manages not to look too heavy on the skin and gives Chanel's Perfection Lumiere Foundation a run for its money.

Beauty decoded: Blotting sheets

Blotting sheets are oily skin's saviour. Re-applying powder more than once can give skin that overdone, cloggy look. Dabbing a blotting sheet, available from high-end to budget brands, on oily patches magically restores balance to the face and eliminates shine. The sheet absorbs the oil while leaving the pigment behind, so you're not taking off half your make-up every time you blot. It works in an instant, but will prolong the staying power of your make-up by a couple of hours at least.

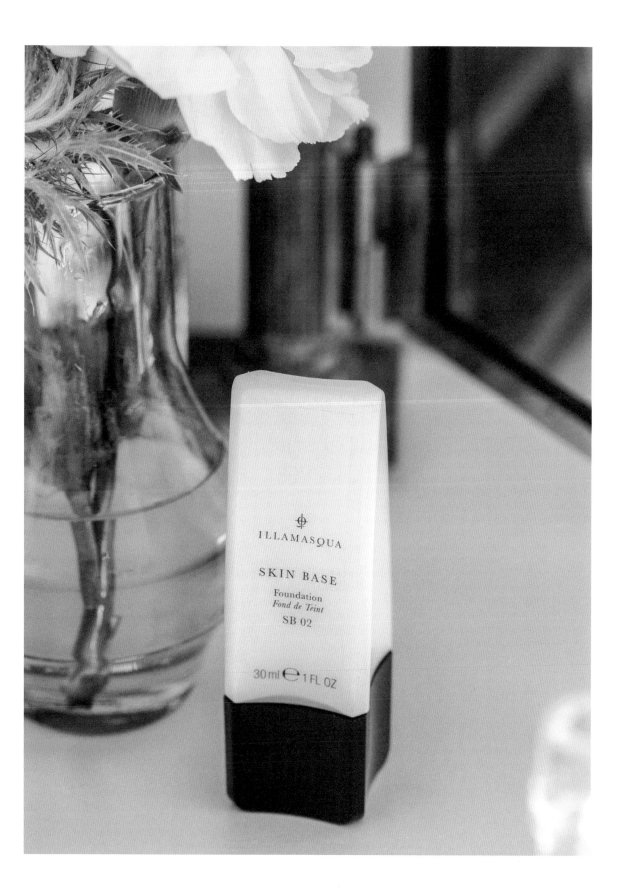

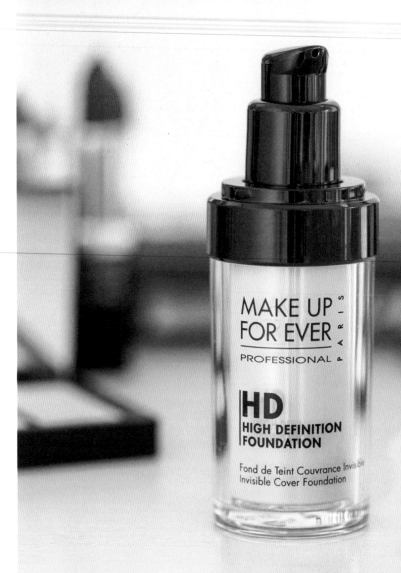

BEST LIGHT COVERAGE

For oilier skins, lighter and more moisturising formulations can be harder to wear. If you still crave the barely-there lightness but don't want to have to powder yourself half to death, then the cult classic Laura Mercier Tinted Moisturiser is oil-free. It comes in several versions depending on your skin type, with a nice shade range and a reliable reputation. Like an old friend we regularly visit, we're very fond of it.

Sisley Phyto Teint Expert Foundation is a quality foundation that blends evenly and stays fresh-looking for the entire day. The liquid-to-powder formula also manages to magically fill in pores, leaving skin looking smooth and even. Applied minimally, it provides light-to-medium coverage that does not feel heavy or dry, but it is quite matte. Yes, it costs a fortune but come hail, rain or snow this will not budge, and, as it is oil-free, it is ideal for normal, combination and oily skin.

Nars Pure Radiant Tinted Moisturizer has been around for a while, but it boasts that cleverness that seems unique to Nars products. The coverage is nice and the shade range impressive, while the finish behaves like a foundation with all the breathability of a silk veil over the face.

Clinique Even Better Makeup is a nice oil-free option for those prone to breakthrough shine during the day. Easily applied with clean fingers, it's a good option for oily or slightly problematic skin. For a more affordable option, try L'Oréal Nude Magique Eau de Teint Fresh Feel Foundation. It's wonderfully light and glowy without being overly damp on the skin.

Beauty decoded: HD foundations

HD foundations have become ever more popular with the advent of HD television. Essentially, HD TV is pretty unforgiving and actresses who had previously looked inhumanly perfect on camera suddenly started to look more like everyone else. The horror.

HD foundations blur fine lines and blemishes more than a standard foundation because they contain ingredients like mica and silicone that have a blurring effect and encourage light to bounce off the skin, creating a smoother and more perfect-looking base.

This all sounds very tempting, but seriously how many of us are on telly every day and need to be camera-ready at all times? That's right, none. Well, Jean Byrne maybe, but she can do what she likes because she is fabulous. A HD foundation won't ever save you from the grey light of a Limerick morning in October or the stark light of a Wexford afternoon in July.

Some HD foundations, like Make Up For Ever HD Invisible Cover Foundation and Revlon PhotoReady Makeup, are wearable in real life (and look great too) but they tend to offer heavier coverage, so are best left for night-time shenanigans. Others, like Smashbox Liquid Halo HD Foundation, are lighter and more feasible as everyday foundation options.

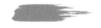

DRY SKIN

Dry skin can be a real pain – sometimes literally. It can chap, it's prone to eczema and rosacea and it's the hardest skin type to apply make-up over. Though dry or flaky skin is something all of us are prone to at certain times of the year or during certain activities (deep-sea fishermen, you have our sympathies), some of us – like Aisling – are just naturally prone to it. That's unfortunate but it's far from a life sentence to flakiness without parole. There's so much that you can do to tackle it so that you have the best possible canvas for foundation.

First off, make sure that your skin is in fact dry and not just dehydrated (page 83). Skin can actually be oily and dehydrated at the same time, so if you're staring at the mirror with dangerous levels of rage and bafflement at the fact that you have flakiness on your oily t-zone, never fear. Your skin is dehydrated. Drink more water and apply a great hydrating serum like Hydraluron Moisture Booster from Indeed Labs with a hydrating moisturiser at bed time. If you're particularly dehydrated or flaky, try applying a hydrating mask like Clinique Moisture Surge Overnight Mask and leave it for ten minutes before cleansing and putting on your foundation. This will hydrate the skin and prepare it perfectly for your base, minimising patchiness and plumping everything nicely.

If you're classically dry, then your skin is underproducing oil so getting yourself in debt to Irish Water won't help a jot. What you need is a lovely facial oil. If you're truly dry-skinned, try applying something like Clarins Blue Orchid Face Treatment Oil underneath make-up to make your complexion sing with radiance. Just give it ten or so minutes to allow it to sink in to your skin before applying foundation, or your make-up might move a little.

Once you've prepped your skin, the foundation options for dry skin are pretty much endless.

If you're classically dry, then your skin is under-producing oil so getting yourself in debt to Irish Water won't help a jot. What you need is a lovely facial oil.

*The ultimate proof that a product is a winner is being
asked by people in admiring tones, 'What foundation/
eyeliner/mascara are you wearing?'*

BEST MEDIUM COVERAGE

Mac Face and Body Foundation is the make-up artist's choice for editorial and catwalk work. You'll rarely see an orange model because make-up artists apply this to limbs as well as faces for perfectly shade-matched coverage. No corned beef legs here. The film fixer in this formula makes it thicken on contact with the air, so apply it immediately for super-light coverage or leave it to sit for two minutes on the back of your hand and you'll have medium-coverage foundation. The shade range is enormous and this flatters dry skin like nothing else.

By Terry Cover-Expert Perfecting Fluid Foundation offers very buildable coverage with a deliciously glowy finish that looks great on drier skins. It's a particularly good 'special occasion' foundation, partially because it's quite expensive, but also because it always makes you look your best.

The coverage of Max Factor Skin Luminizer Foundation is on the full side of medium: it covers everything and you won't need any concealer with it. It has a slightly tacky feel and does settle into fine lines over time, but to up the glow factor, mix it with a brightening CC cream.

Rimmel Match Perfection Foundation is a budget wonder. A dead ringer for YSL's Le Teint Touche Éclat Foundation, it glides on like a dream, leaves the perfect dewy finish, and stays put. Bourjois Healthy Mix Serum, which a lot of people find too greasy, is perfect for dry skin. Dry skin will soak up this gel base and you can just use powder over it if you feel shiny as the day wears on. It provides good coverage and can be built up easily.

The ultimate proof that a product is a winner is being asked by people in admiring tones, 'What foundation/eyeliner/mascara are you wearing?' Clarins Skin Illusion Foundation will get you those compliments. Aisling's absolute favourite, it provides smooth, creamy coverage and plenty of radiance.

BEST LIGHT COVERAGE

Chantecaille Just Skin Tinted Moisturizer certainly isn't a budget wonder, but it is pretty wondrous. Inspired by Japanese bases, which place greater emphasis on foundation's skincare potential than Western products, this is more of a tinted moisturiser than a foundation, but it perfects skin to leave it looking healthy and refreshed. Add a touch of concealer to cover blemishes and you'll have flawless skin in no time.

Estée Lauder Perfectionist Youth-Infusing Makeup is another of Aisling's favourite foundations. She's been hooked since the first time she tried it, which was one of those mornings from hell. It was applied in a hasty and slapdash manner, but resulted in a finish that was flawless, looked lustrous and reflected light. It lasted well all day, felt as hydrating as a moisturiser and just needed a touch-up around her nose later in the afternoon. This is light-to-medium coverage that looks polished and expensive and disguises the look of lines, but it is not suitable for bad skin days. If you like this foundation, you'll also love Artistry Youth XTend Lifting Smoothing Foundation, which provides perfect, lightweight coverage.

Giorgio Armani Luminous Silk Foundation is completely iconic for a reason. Radiant on the skin, it is buildable to just about medium coverage, but is at its best applied lightly for healthy, glowing skin. Another innovative offering from Giorgio Armani, its Crema Nuda Supreme Glow Reviving Tinted Cream, works well for all skin types, but is particularly at home on dry skin. Armani are pitching this fabulously heavy jar of complexion perfector as a cross between a luxury BB and a CC cream. The coverage is light but can be built to medium, and the choice of six shades means you can choose one to give you a summer-kissed glow while the hydrating benefits of the cream will keep your skin feeling fresh.

To refresh foundation that's starting to look a bit dry and settled after a few hours' wear, whip out a facial spritz – Mac Prep+Prime Fix+ is a nice one – and liberally spritz your face. It will refresh your make-up and your spirits.

Beauty tip: Combination skin and foundation

Almost everyone is prone to slight oiliness in certain areas and at certain ages. This doesn't mean that you have two opposing skin types. If you still have a tendency to be very oily in one part of the face but dry in another, then the only option – unfortunately – is to wear two foundations, or to wear an oil-absorbing primer where you are prone to oiliness. Experiment with different formulations, and you will find what makes your skin happiest.

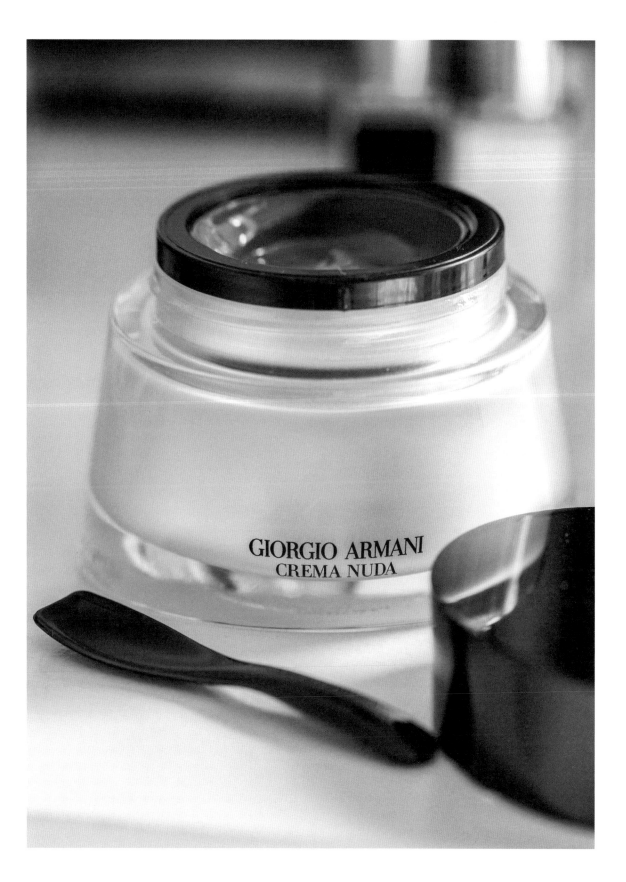

ACNE-PRONE SKIN

People can be unfairly dismissive of acne, particularly if the sufferer is a teenager. But no one has the right to dictate what should or should not affect your self-esteem, what you should 'get over' or 'put up with'. Rather than feeling bad about yourself and possibly worsening the acne by smothering it with heavy foundations, instead choose a base that won't look caked on and use concealer to cover the blemishes. Also resist the temptation to drench it in alcohol-laden acne products. Instead pare back your skincare routine, re-evaluate and if your acne is acute enough, ask for a referral to a dermatologist. Make-up is no replacement for confidence or happiness in your own skin.

When we think of oily and acne-prone skin, we generally think of teens, but the highest rate of diagnoses of acne is, interestingly, in women over forty. You've already gone through the hormonal hell-train that is puberty, and now you find your hormones buggering your skin once again. It can be unbelievably frustrating.

Obviously, topical products can't fix a hormonal imbalance, but while you try to get your skin back on track, there are some clever, hard-working foundations that can help to restore your sense of control a little. We completely understand the urge to go full throttle and apply the heaviest coverage you can get your hands on, but unless your acne is in the top 5% of severity, you will still have patches of clear, healthy skin around the face and neck. By allowing these to show through but carefully concealing the acne, you're keeping the focus on the best parts of your skin, which will make the overall finish more like natural-looking skin and less like masses of foundation.

Vichy Dermablend Corrective Foundation is the classic choice as it can cover any pigmentation from acne to birth marks. We suggest

When we think of oily and acne-prone skin, we generally think of teens, but the highest rate of diagnoses of acne is, interestingly, in women over forty.

*Our national love affair with full-coverage
foundation shows no signs of abating.*

that you use this full-coverage foundation as a concealer rather than applying it all over the face. For everywhere else, opt for a lighter base. Anything designed for oily skin (page 125) should work nicely, but remember to allow your skin to show through – it's the blemishes that we want to cover.

If you really only feel comfortable wearing a full-coverage foundation, or full coverage is just what you most like, Mac Full Coverage Foundation is serious stuff. This is an incredibly thick compact formulation, so thick in fact that it's best applied with a damp sponge and patted on in thin layers. There's no messing with this stuff – it is the most complete coverage foundation outside of professional and special effects products from brands like Kryolan that we've encountered. It does the job, but it certainly doesn't feel light on the skin. Though it works fantastically as a concealer, wearing the waxy formula all over may not do any favours for acne-prone skin.

Clinique Beyond Perfecting Foundation + Concealer will cover everything, while Revlon

Colorstay Makeup for Normal/Dry Skin is another great option. And there's no way we could discuss full-coverage foundations without giving an honorary mention to Estée Lauder Double Wear Stay-in-Place Makeup, which is now available in a handy travel compact. The Irish woman's full coverage go-to for decades now, our national love affair with it doesn't seem to be abating. If you want something tried and tested that will conceal everything in sight, this is for you. Beware, though: unless you go very lightly, it will look heavy on the skin. Choose Estée Lauder Double Wear Light Stay-in-Place Makeup if you want to take it down a notch as it still provides plenty of coverage.

If you want to go lighter on the coverage but still use something acne-appropriate, the Clinique Anti-Blemish Solutions Liquid Makeup is a winner. The lightweight formula feels nice on the skin, but still offers substantial coverage. It's formulated to neutralise redness and discolouration, so it's a good choice if acne scarring is a concern.

~~~~~~~~~

A primer is a good idea if you find that your foundation has a tendency to wander and settle in places.

~~~~~~~~~

MATURE SKIN

Mature skin varies just like skin at every other age, but generally the skin needs more moisture and benefits most from radiant formulations and softer, more forgiving textures. Matte finishes tend to sink into mature skin, highlighting lines and leaving a tired-looking complexion that absorbs light rather than reflecting it.

Provided the skin is happy (see 'Mature skin', page 86, for tips on a comprehensive skincare regime that can make a visible difference), start by taking a good look at what your skin is doing before deciding on what type of foundation to use.

A primer is a good idea if you find that your foundation has a tendency to wander and settle in places. This will help its lasting power too. Moist formulations act best and you can always set any shinier areas with a touch of powder after you've applied your foundation.

No7 Instant Radiance Foundation takes after bases like YSL's famous Le Teint Touche Éclat Foundation. Glowy and radiant, it applies equally well with a brush or with fingers.

YSL Youth Liberator Serum Foundation is a specifically targeted pro-ageing foundation that has all the might of YSL's impressive shade range behind it. Light in texture but comfortingly smooth, it offers medium buildable coverage and lasts nicely on the skin.

Bobbi Brown Intensive Skin Serum Foundation is a seriously good foundation. Though it works for younger skins too, mature skin will benefit from the almost syrupy yet breathable formula and formidable coverage.

If your skin is mature but you like something very light and barely-there-looking that evens out the complexion without looking like make-up, though pricey Crème De La Mer Reparative Skintint is a beauty. This is fresh-faced minimalism at its very best.

Clarins Extra-Comfort Foundation is the perfect medium-coverage option for mature skin, which needs something a little richer and more forgiving. A thick unctuous goo, it applies equally nicely with fingers or a brush and feels softly soothing on the skin. Just don't eat it.

If you're more mature or have dry skin and your concern is finish rather than coverage, then Bobbi Brown Extra SPF 25 Tinted Moisturizing Balm is perfect. Ultra-light and leaving a radiant finish on the skin, it's an effort-free good skin day in a tub.

Beauty decoded: Mineral foundation

We sometimes encounter make-up enthusiasts who will only wear powder foundations, claiming that they're purer and better for the skin than alternatives. The truth is that this isn't always true.

Certainly, the mineral pigments in foundations like bareMinerals Original Foundation and Clarins Skin Illusion Loose Powder Foundation are too large to be absorbed by the skin, and so they sit atop it pretty harmlessly while giving you some nice coverage. But it's also the case that mineral foundations often contain other ingredients like rice powder, which is a talc substitute and actually very nice, especially as an oil absorber for a matte finish, but it's hardly a mineral.

Although we associate mineral foundations with powder formulas, they're available in all forms, including liquid. It's just a matter of doing your research and choosing the formula that's best for you, with the finish you're most fond of. Mineral powder foundations are sort of a love/hate product. Lots of people adore the matte finish and easy application, while others find them drab-looking and prone to sitting in dry patches.

If you'd like a mineral foundation but have dry skin, opt for a liquid version like Mac Mineralize Moisture Foundation. It has a soft, glowy finish but is still a mineral foundation. Mineral foundations are much more widely and cheaply available in powder form; No7 Mineral Perfection Powder Foundation is a nice option.

Finally, don't be fooled by the SPF claims of powder foundations. Though they do contain titanium dioxide and other physical sunblocks, they don't contain sufficient quantities to properly protect your skin. Apply a separate SPF underneath for better protection. Mineral foundations are handy to have in the handbag, but they're not a cure-all product.

Mineral powder foundations are sort of a love/hate product. Lots of people adore the matte finish and easy application, while others find them drab-looking and prone to sitting in dry patches.

FOUNDATIONS FOR PALE SKIN

After years in hiding (mostly under a thick coating of orange goo), fair-skinned women have finally begun to embrace their natural paleness. Unfortunately, because many fair *cailíns* spent so long trying to use foundation to morph themselves into another ethnicity, lots of brands don't provide a comprehensive range of paler shades for lily-white women, because they haven't been buying them. Even some brands that were traditionally a pale girl's best friend, like Bobbi Brown, have discontinued their palest shades in some of their lines – Bobbi Brown's Alabaster is now only available in some formulations.

The only way to bring them back is to increase demand. The more fair-skinned women embrace their naturally fair skin, the more beauty brands will start to provide the right products to do justice by it.

It's hard to have confidence in bossy make-up counter assistants declaring that pale-skinned people need something three shades deeper than their natural skin colour to 'warm them up'. No one needs to be warmed up. And even if they did, 'warming up' isn't a thing. What fair-skinned women need is a product that won't leave them with a tideline along their jaw or oxidise into a violent orange as soon as they leave the make-up counter and go outside into the world.

If you'd like to look like you've taken some sun, then what you need is a foundation that matches the colour of your natural skin and a really good bronzer. You'll look sun-kissed and glowing, not 'warmed up' like old reheated milk. If you have a very fair complexion, anaemic as the inside of a raw potato, then embrace it. Pale is beautiful.

Although Aisling isn't the palest, (she's halfway between Mac NW15 and NW20), Laura is and she's spent years searching and custom-mixing foundation shades to find foundations that aren't just pale enough, but also the right undertone, so that there's no horrible yellow, grey or overly pink caste to them. None of them, ever, have been called 'toasty beige'.

If you have a very pale complexion, then the words 'toasty beige' don't apply to you. Leave them to those lucky tanned people and get reacquainted with what you've got. After all, in some countries, looking as milk-bottle white as a parish camogie team playing in November is the epitome of beautiful. If you're pale-skinned, be proud of it. A foundation that matches your skin, regardless of the shade, always makes you look better than one which doesn't.

Estée Lauder Double Wear Light Stay-in-Place Makeup in 1.0 comes from a bigger shade range than any other brand – forty-three and counting. It's no wonder that this much-loved base is a perfect match for pale folk.

Lancôme Teint Miracle Foundation in 010 is light, long-wearing coverage that stays looking fresh throughout the day. All of the Lancôme foundations have good matches for pale skin tones. They seem to understand skin with pink undertones. Though Illamasqua isn't available from make-up counters in Ireland any more,

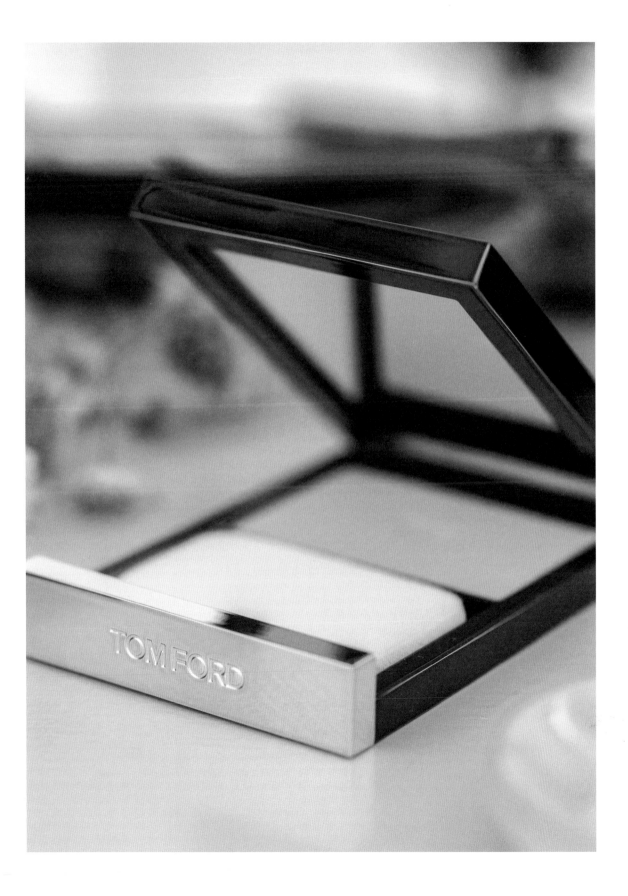

you can find it on Debenhams.ie and the brand's own website. Illamasqua Skin Base Foundation in 02 is make-up artists' favourite and provides a professional smooth base. It cancels out any undertones and comes in several shades of super-pale as well as a very useful white version for lightening your other foundations.

YSL Le Teint Touche Éclat Foundation in B10/ BR10 is a glorious skin day in a bottle and has a pale shade for both yellow and pink undertones. While it's dewy, oilier skin can still get away with it; this really is a pale skin all-rounder.

L'Oréal Infallible Stay Fresh Foundation in Porcelain is comparable to more expensive bases and is available in both pink and yellow tones. It can be tough to find pale shades from budget brands, as they produce fewer options and are motivated by what sells in the largest numbers.

Finally, Nars Sheer Glow Foundation in Siberia is great for those who like a sheer glowy finish that can be built to medium or full coverage. The undertone is decidedly yellow though, so those on the pinker side of pale should avoid it.

If you'd like to look like you've taken some sun, then what you need is a foundation that matches the colour of your natural skin and a really good bronzer.

Bargain beauty: Expensive shade mistakes

Sometimes, despite your best efforts, mistakes are made. You choose the wrong shade of foundation and you find yourself at home attempting to apply a luxury foundation to your face while trying to ignore the fact that it's making you look like an orang-utan.

Ideally, you'd return the foundation and swap it for a perfect match. When this isn't possible, there are a couple of things you can do.

Firstly (and most cost-effectively), you can transform it into a tinted moisturiser. If the colour is only a couple of shades too dark, then combining it with your day moisturiser will tone down the shade. That said, it will also significantly dilute the coverage, so if you want to maintain that, then you may have to make another investment.

If the foundation is too dark but the right undertone, then it's as simple as adding some white foundation on the back of your hand and mixing yourself the right shade. Just keep swatching it along your jawline in order to figure out when you've got the shade just right.

While you can't get Mac Studio Face and Body Foundation in White in Ireland, you can buy it in other countries so if you're keen to get your hands on it, stock up abroad or get a pal to pick up a bottle for you. Mac's website doesn't ship to Ireland, but you could set yourself up with a Parcel Motel account.

Face Atelier Ultra Foundation Pro, available online, comes in a white shade called Zero Minus, which you can mix with foundations to lighten them. It isn't cheap, but it will rescue your mismatched purchase and put it to good use on your face, where it belongs.

If the foundation you've found yourself stuck with is too light, head to that drawer of random foundations you don't use (we all have a drawer full of poorly thought-out purchases) and see if there are any in there you can mix in to deepen the shade. (Or even better, host a swap-shop beauty-product evening at home and swap the foundation with a grateful friend.) Provided the darker shade has the same undertone as the foundation you want to mix it with, it will work nicely. Again, just keep doing the jawline swatch test to check when you've got the match right.

Always mix the foundation on the back of your hand each time you need to apply it. Combining different foundations in bottles may affect their lasting power or cause the formulas to react badly with one another and will end up another expensive mistake.

If the depth of the shade is right but the undertone isn't, the same shade in the opposite undertone should neutralise the colour enough to make it wearable.

If you have somehow ended up with a foundation that is both the wrong shade and undertone, you're pretty much stuck. You would have to mix so many different products into it that it really wouldn't be the original foundation any more. Cut your losses and start over.

FOUNDATIONS FOR DARK SKIN

While 'Irish skin' used to refer solely to the sort of skin you'd see on the bacon-hued legs of GAA players in short shorts during the '70s, the phrase has expanded to include all kinds and shades of skin. Irish women now boast a kaleidoscope of skin colours and tones and thankfully make-up brands here are starting to respond and cater to the needs of women of various skin tones and shades. It's about time.

Where paler skins often suffer from redness, darker skins tend towards greyness and the products to counteract this are very different. Women with dark skin tones sometimes need two different shades of foundation on different areas of their face, as darker skin can vary more in pigment, but there are several great foundation options.

Darker skins have yellow or red undertones – if you have dark skin, your perfect match will mimic your natural undertone. Match it to the skin on your chest area rather than the face for a flawless match. The chest is the largest expanse of skin likely to be displayed, so matching the face to the skin in this area creates a uniform, natural-looking finish. Always match in daylight, as department store lighting is a notorious liar.

Bobbi Brown Skin Foundation Stick works for normal to dry skin and the darkest shade, Espresso, has a very subtle sparkle that gives a beautiful glow. Darker skins reflect the light better than pale skins do, so products with shimmer and highlight in them look divinely radiant on the skin and give it extra definition. Mac Studio Sculpt Foundation is creamy and radiant, giving a beautiful dewy finish. It's available in a wide range of colours from pale to dark. Giorgio Armani Luminous Silk Foundation is one of the best foundations on the market and the shades for darker skin are beautiful. Debenhams have a range specifically for black skin, called black|Up, which is very popular. Their Full Coverage Cream Foundation is great for women who like complete coverage with a comfy finish.

Pharmacy brands in Ireland haven't caught up with department store brands in catering for either dark or very pale skin. The palest and darkest skins are sometimes excluded, which is maddening. Women with darker skin are often left with just one or two shade options, neither of which are the right one for them, when shopping for cheaper foundations. Darker skins vary more in shade than lighter skins do, so it's time for more brands to reflect this. Like the super-pale, people with darker skin often have to spend that bit more to find their right match and they shouldn't have to.

Beauty tip: When foundations oxidise

If you've noticed that your lovely new foundation goes orange or turns a few shades darker after a while on your face, it has oxidised. This is incredibly frustrating and happens mostly to oily-skinned people when the combination of your skin's natural oils and oxygen in the atmosphere react with certain ingredients in your foundation to darken it.

There's not a huge amount that you can do to counteract this – it's generally a sign that the foundation isn't up to standard. If it's new, you should feel totally entitled to return it.

The WTF of Alphabet Creams

It's no secret in the cosmetics world that Alphabet Creams saved the industry from the recession. The original East–West beauty hybrid, BB creams were the original Asian import and their arrival was greeted with great excitement by cosmetic companies and consumers alike. We all thought, '*Oh how nice. Something really different. That's refreshing*', and hurried to buy the products.

Every brand zealously set about to convince women that they needed these creams: they peeled the stickers off their existing tinted moisturiser products and renamed them BB creams, they added foundation to day moisturisers and in short they deliberately confused the life out of consumers. Naturally, people wanted to try these new products. They sometimes bought several different types and became puzzled by the differences between brands and the inconsistency in formulation. Cash registers continued to ring as we all tried to find the perfect BB cream for us – it was cha-ching time for the cosmetic industry.

In 2013 Euromonitor warned the beauty industry against the overuse of the term 'BB cream' as it had moved so far from the original Asian concept that the Western versions, by and large, bore no similarity to the original products. Consumers were being deliberately misled by these products, which promised so many multi-functional benefits that some of them only stopped short of promising to hang out the washing and make you a cup of tea when you got in from work. We've since raced past CC and DD and we're now on to EE and FF – and if we ever get on to GG, we'll go utterly bonkers.

Resist the temptation to pull your hair out and bellow your demands for justice at the sky. The alphabet monikers are more tired than an exhausted shopper determinedly trying to climb up the down escalator so the best way to navigate this domain of alphabetised products is to forget about the names and judge them based on formulation. If you're interested in buying one, check what it's promising (world domination probably, but a cursory go on the Google machine will help with that) and then see if it delivers when you test it. It's as simple as that.

The best way to navigate this domain of alphabetised products is to forget about the names and judge them based on formulation.

BB CREAMS

Though we're all thoroughly exhausted by the bombardment of letters and it feels as though they've been around forever, BB creams actually made their first appearance as a Westernised product in 2012. Though they were inspired by Asian, and particularly Korean BB creams, the Western version is quite different.

BB is an acronym of 'Beauty Balm', and the original Korean iteration was heavily focused on light coverage combined with impressive skincare, because Asian women have a strong reputation for being very serious about their skincare. The idea was to care for skin while also acting as a base, in a way that products hadn't done before. Asian BB creams offer much wider shade ranges and feel quite different in texture.

Western versions are more along the lines of a tinted moisturiser and vary widely in terms of the quality of skincare components. They tend to come in limited shade ranges, which is far from ideal, although some of them are lovely as light bases, particularly during the summer, when you're in the mood to wear less make-up.

Smashbox Camera Ready BB Cream is a nice option. Thicker than standard BB creams and with coverage that can be built up to medium, it is slightly more like a light foundation than a BB cream. Kiehl's Skin Tone Correcting & Beautifying BB Cream is more along the lines of its Asian counterparts. Featuring SPF 50 and free of mineral oil, this one is a winner if you can find a shade-match.

If you like something with a very soft but slightly thicker texture, L'Occitane Precious BB Cream is a good bet if you can find a shade-match from its limited range of three shades.

We think that Mac Prep+Prime Beauty Balm is very underrated. Perfect for Mac's chief demographic of younger people with oily skin, it comes in eight shades and creates a dewy complexion that somehow stays put on oily skin. Rimmel BB Cream Radiance is a beautifully glowy option at under a tenner, but it's only available in three shades.

BB creams generally don't cater for people on either end of the skin tone spectrum so they are pretty useless for the palest- and darkest-skinned beauty enthusiasts, who have to opt for a tinted moisturiser or light foundation instead.

And when BB creams for hair were launched? Well, we nearly lost the will to live.

BB is an acronym of 'Beauty Balm', and the original Korean iteration was heavily focused on light coverage combined with impressive skincare, because Asian women have a strong reputation for being very serious about their skincare.

CC CREAMS

After BB came CC. Meaning 'colour correction', CC creams use colour theory, which is the idea that opposing hues on the colour wheel can be used to counteract one another, a guiding principle taught to all professional make-up artists, and neutralise pigmentation issues without looking heavy on the skin.

Aimed at people with redness, under-eye darkness or general pigmentation issues and patchiness, these products frequently do live up to their hype. They generally contain tiny particles of various tints and colours that act to conceal discolouration and they tend to work well. Obviously, any extreme discolouration needs concealer, but for the more everyday redness, blueness and greyness that we're all prone to, these will do the job.

Bourjois 123 Perfect CC Cream offers very impressive coverage for a product that looks so unassuming in the tube and is slightly runny in consistency. Again, shades are limited, but if you can find yours, it's definitely worth trying.

For more mature skin, Chanel Complete Correction CC Cream is beautiful. Dewier and less oil-absorbent than the Bourjois 123 Perfect CC Cream, the thick consistency melts on contact with the skin for a finish that glows.

YSL Forever Light Creator CC Cream is gorgeous. You can wear it under foundation or on its own and it will actually make your skin glow. Clinique Moisture Surge CC Cream is another nice option, though it can settle into dry skin despite the name, so moisturise well before you apply it.

Aimed at people with redness, under-eye darkness or general pigmentation issues and patchiness, CC creams frequently do live up to their hype.

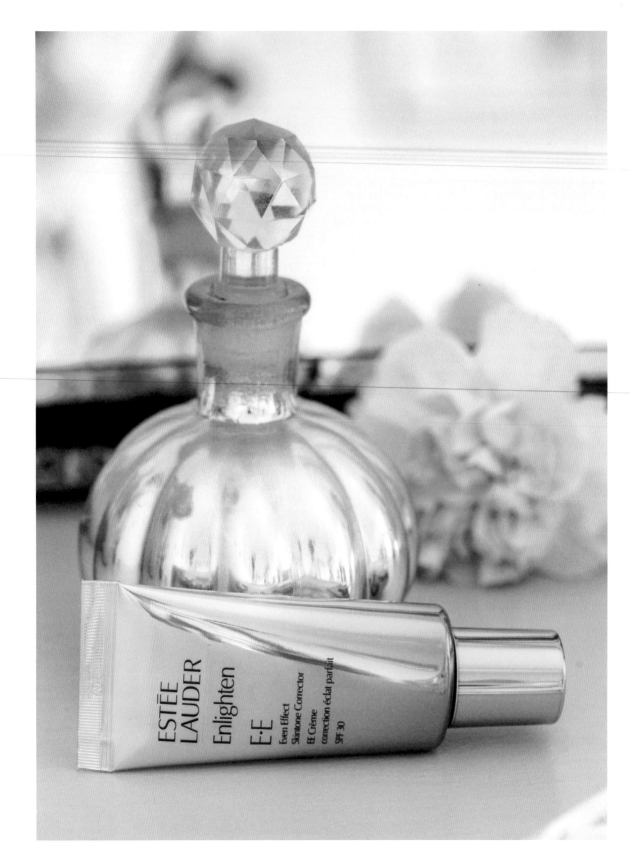

The agony continues. BB creams in their original Asian form were great, CC creams do genuinely help to act as colour correctors. But DD creams? At this point, we're just tired.

DD CREAMS

The agony continues. BB creams in their original Asian form were great, CC creams do genuinely help to act as colour correctors. But DD creams? At this point, we're just tired.

DD creams claim to combine the tint and skincare benefits of a BB with the colour-correcting clout of a CC and offer defence while they're at it. Some companies refer to DD creams as 'Dynamic Do-all' and some claim that the acronym DD stands for 'Daily Defence' but frankly, BB and CC creams both offer defence in the form of SPF, so we don't really feel the need for DD creams.

The idea that this is an all-in-one product that dispenses with the need for any skincare underneath is just nonsense. Some DD creams, like Nuxe Crème Prodigieuse DD Crème, are quite nice but they're really best as tinted moisturisers more than anything else. Calm down, beauty industry. You're trying too hard.

EE CREAMS

At this point, we're tempted to dispense with the whole alphabet and just head to the pub because it's getting beyond ridiculous, and every new Alphabet Cream seems to be a combination of the previous ones repackaged as something new.

In 2014 Estée Lauder launched the first EE cream, which they called Enlighten Even Effect Skintone Corrector. It claims to treat, rather than just cover like a CC cream, pigmentation spots caused by sun damage. It is a really nice light foundation. But that's what it is: a foundation.

In short, just no. Go home, foundation, you're drunk.

CHAPTER 12

· CONCEALER ·

We're make-up obsessives: obsessed with make-up in general, with our own ever-expanding collections and with the contents of other people's make-up bags. And we love that when we ask women what make-up product they'd rather not be without, the one that they would never want to part with, there's generally no agreement. The product that makes you feel most ready to face the world in the morning is different for everyone.

For Laura, that product is concealer. She admits that her love of it probably stems from the days when she suffered badly with acne and felt that concealer helped to restore her self-confidence and sense of control over her own face when the acne made her feel powerless and vulnerable.

Though a careful skincare routine has helped to regulate her skin enormously – it occasionally misbehaves, but not too much these days – her resounding love of concealer has remained. There's less to cover up, but she still loves concealer just as much.

Concealer is designed to cover blemishes. Many of us make the mistake of just using very heavy foundation to do this, when we don't need to. A light base looks more like real skin. Instead, use a great concealer to disguise any imperfections. That way your make-up will look more like perfect skin.

Choosing your concealer colour

Kim Kardashian has a fierce amount to answer for. She's brought contouring, which was originally a stage and drag make-up trick, a visual illusion that really only works in certain light and from a certain distance, into the world of everyday make-up. She's also standardised the use of a number of concealer shades at the same time to highlight facial structure and create a completely flawless complexion.

In a way, that's great. She has inspired a generation of people to enjoy make-up and express themselves, so we suppose we can't hold her personally responsible for every set of orange speed stripes we see scrawled on the side of people's faces or for the people who use make-up to try to express Kim Kardashian rather than themselves.

The lighter your skin tone, the less variation in natural shade it exhibits (unless you count redness, which we generally try to cover rather than enhance). Dark skins are a make-up artist's dream because they catch and reflect light and shadow in a much more dramatic way. Women with dark skin tones are more prone to varied skin tone in certain areas of their face than very pale-skinned women and have been using lighter concealers and foundations in the centre of their faces for a long time, but that particular practice seems to have evaded us here in Éire until pretty recently.

Still, if you're pale-skinned, don't despair. Pale-skinned women can learn a lot from the make-up techniques traditionally used by women of colour – concealer can be used not only to conceal, but to add dimension to the face. You can use concealers of varying colours to give your face dimension if you're paler; you just can't vary the shades as dramatically as someone with darker skin can without looking a bit odd.

When choosing a concealer, opt for one up to two shades lighter than your normal skin tone if you're planning to use it under your eyes. More than this, and your face will start to look imbalanced.

You should also stick to the two-shade rule if you're using concealer to contour – if you go more than two shades deeper than the shade of your skin, you'll have to spend an age blending and the effect won't look convincing in daylight.

If you're opting for a natural look that mirrors your make-up-free skin at its very best, just match your concealer to your natural skin tone. To find the right shade, swatch it along your jawline just as you would with foundation. The shade that disappears is your perfect match.

Applying concealer

Skin is more disloyal than your first boyfriend, who may or may not have broken up with you via a text that read 'Dis nt wrkn. Soz'. If he didn't, he certainly had the emotional capacity to and you know it.

The minute your life gets in any way difficult (which, let's face it, is rather often), your skin mutinies like a ship full of scurvy-ridden pirates who've decided to knock the captain down a peg or two.

Skin: '*Oh, you haven't had much sleep, have you? That's terrible. I'll just make you look plague-ridden so you remember to go to bed early, okay?*'

You: '*Um …*'

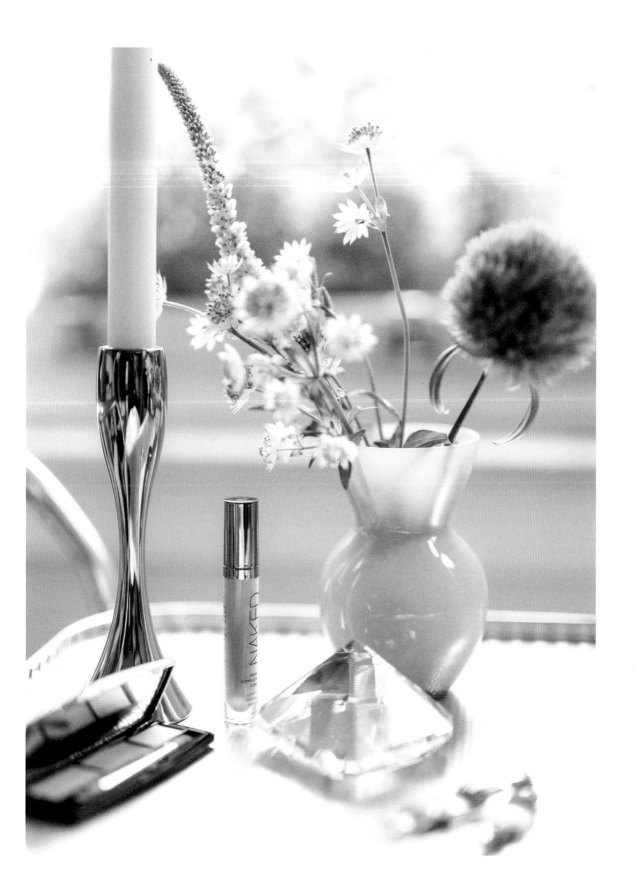

Skin: *'Oh, you've been busy and not eating well? I understand, no problem. Here's a chin boil. Don't do it again.'*

You: *'Oh for the love of ...'*

Like an unwieldy toddler, your skin requires constant attention and reassurance and when it doesn't get it, it throws itself on the supermarket floor and starts wailing inconsolably about biscuits. Concealer will tamp down your skin's shrieks while you get it back into a disciplined routine and end its reign of terror.

The key to great make-up is perfecting your base. No matter how accomplished your smoky eye is, if your base isn't even and applied well, the overall effect is going to look sloppy. So although fingers always work brilliantly, we think that a brush specifically for concealer is a sound investment because it gives a buffed effect that fingers can't achieve on their own. It doesn't have to be a designated 'concealer brush'. It can be any brush that works for you and achieves the finish you prefer.

The Setting Brush by Real Techniques is one of our favourite brushes. It's a fantastic little multitasker. Originally intended for setting make-up under the eyes with powder, we like it for buffing liquid concealer over dark circles for an airbrushed finish. Laura has two, and keeps one in her handbag at all times alongside her beloved Nars Radiant Creamy Concealer in case she needs to sweep some under her eyes or cover one of those sudden violent blemishes you only ever seem to get when you leave the house. This brilliant brush buffs concealer (and foundation, if you have the time and the inclination) seamlessly. In a fix, you could even use it to blend your eyeshadow.

This is a particularly nice and affordable brush, but any synthetic fluffy brush will do. With a brush that you use several times a day (if you use the same one for touch-ups when you're out and about) frequent washing is essential (page 158), particularly if your skin is prone to breaking out. Synthetic brushes tend to absorb less product, wash more easily and dry quicker than natural hair.

Concealing blemishes like spots and scars can be tricky business. For the fiddly work and pin-point concealing of little blemishes, you should opt for a fine brush, like a tiny eyeliner pinpoint brush, or something fluffy but still quite small. Again, Real Techniques knock out high-quality, affordable brushes. Their small Eyeshadow Brush has synthetic fibres that don't absorb much product and the tiny brush-head makes concealing in fiddly areas like under brows or the sides of the nose a breeze. Its fluffy texture blends the edges of your concealer so that it has no definable beginning or end. Yes, a small eyeshadow brush is technically for eyeshadow (it works really well for that too) but brushes try to fulfil any task you put them to, so feel free to stretch their limits. Experiment – you'll soon find an unorthodox favourite that you never thought would cover blemishes so well.

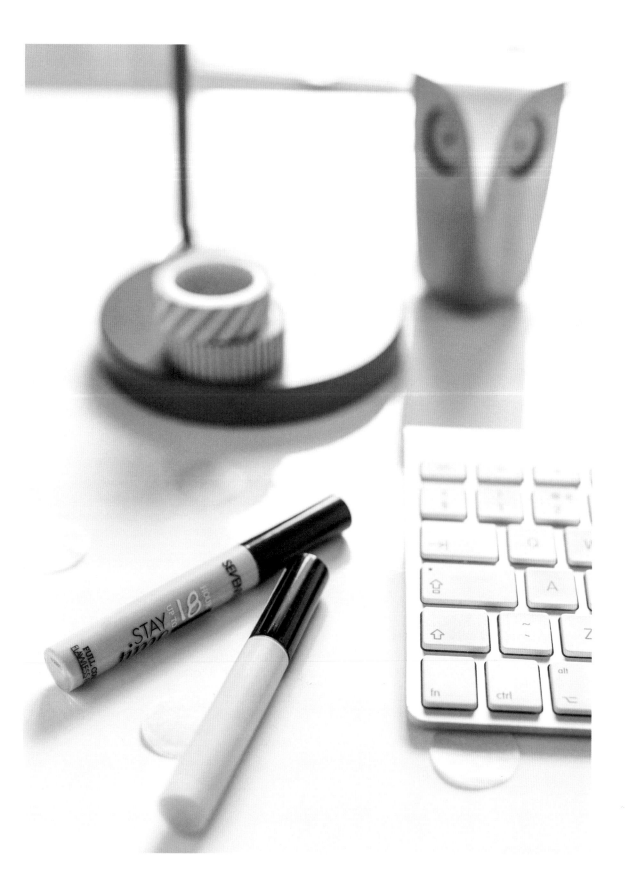

The best concealers

There are three qualities a good concealer must have: excellent coverage, a moist(ish) formulation and an absolutely flawless shade-match for your skin. If your concealer is lighter or darker than your skin, it will draw the eye to a blemish rather than concealing it.

Nars Radiant Creamy Concealer is a cure-all for covering every standard kind of blemish. It does equally well on dark circles and the nastiest blemishes. The shade range is widely inclusive and the thick liquid formula dries down to perfect coverage.

For more conspicuous discolouration, like red scarring, a very opaque concealer is the only thing that will fully camouflage. Kevyn Aucoin The Sensual Skin Enhancer is a professional-quality multitasking product. Combined with moisturiser, it turns into something similar to foundation. Applied straight to the skin, it conceals almost anything. Proceed carefully though, as this is seriously thick and opaque – a very little amount is enough to cover even the angriest or most discoloured blemish.

Mac Select Moisturecover is a more everyday concealer that works well for standard under-eye and blemish cover. The shade range is great and the dewy formulation is great for slightly drier skin.

Collection Lasting Perfection Ultimate Wear Concealer is – in our opinion – the best affordable concealer on the market. Though the shade range is limited, if you can find a match, the coverage is long-lasting and perfect. Seventeen 18 Hour Stay Time Concealer is a great option for dry or more mature skin. It has a slightly dewy consistency which blends seamlessly, can be layered and offers great coverage.

There are three qualities a good concealer must have: excellent coverage, a moist(ish) formulation and an absolutely flawless shade-match for your skin.

You'd think that professionals would be immune to the errors that have the rest of us looking ridiculous in photos, but in a way it's comforting to know that even people who know their stuff can make silly make-up mistakes.

Beauty decoded: Light-reflective concealers

When you see photos of celebrities with that strange ghostly whiteness under their eyes, their make-up artist has made a really common mistake. You'd think that professionals would be immune to the errors that have the rest of us looking ridiculous in photos, but in a way it's comforting to know that even people who know their stuff can make silly make-up mistakes. It's just more unfortunate as when they bugger up, it's on Jennifer Lawrence's face and the photos aren't confined to the album where you keep those photos of you wearing chocolate-brown lipstick while sitting on a stranger's knee back in 1993.

Irish women aren't alone in their habit of misusing light-reflective concealers. We have an awful habit of glancing in the mirror, observing moon eyes sunk into the two blue lagoons that are apparently our eye sockets. We get a fright and rush for anything than has the word 'light' on it, from diet yoghurt to light-reflective concealer.

These products aren't concealers and they don't counteract blueness. YSL Touche Éclat, which is possibly the most iconic light-reflective concealer pen ever, was never intended as a concealer. Instead, it's the ultimate in cosmetic luxury: the pen is beautiful, but it's really a very subtle liquid highlighter.

You might put a tiny dab of powder or liquid highlighter on the inner corner of your eye, but you'd never sweep a load of powder highlighter underneath your eye. It won't cover the blueness, will highlight bags and wrinkles, and will have you looking like a shiny insomniac.

What's more, in photographs, the flash will bounce off the pigments in the highlighter and reflect back towards the camera, creating that weird white effect underneath the eyes that makes you look a bit untidy and crazed.

If you love Touche Éclat or a similar highlighting pen product, you should instead blend it along the top of your cheekbones, down your nose and on your cupid's bow. This will make your bone structure pop in flash photography and ensure that the features you'd rather conceal stay concealed.

CHAPTER 13

· BLUSH ·

For seasoned make-up lovers, blush is a pretty straightforward affair but nothing is simple until you know how to do it, and a lot of women are un-equivocally terrified of blush out of a fear that it will leave them looking clownish. Read on and don't worry – it won't.

Lots of Irish people, both male and female, have a slightly rubicund complexion. Rosacea is far more common here in Ireland (and to a slightly lesser extent in the UK) than it is in warmer climes. The right skincare routine can hugely improve rosacea, but some of us are simply genetically predisposed to ruddiness and no amount of skincare will change that.

Often, women skip blush altogether in an attempt to minimise redness. This is a mistake in almost every case. If you are applying your foundation well, then you're literally blanking out your facial features.

Think of make-up application as an art. The principles of art are dictated by light and shadow. When you apply foundation, you're creating a blank canvas. In order for make-up to look natural and flattering, you must put the light and shadow you've removed with foundation back into the face. If you don't, you will actually look like you're wearing far more make-up than if you add a touch of blush and perhaps some highlighter. Skin with just foundation on it looks like foundation, not skin.

When Laura was in her teens, the frenzy for contouring hadn't hit yet, and girls would apply full-coverage foundation all over their faces (and the lips, too. Never a good look.) before heading off about their day. Blush was an alien concept. The effect was two bizarre-ly overlined eyes winking out of a moonish orange face, frequently with a nasty tideline at the neck where the colour they wanted to be met the colour they actually were. This is a pretty disturbing look. Nobody wants to be scaring small children on their way home from school.

No person's face is entirely one colour, re-gardless of their ethnicity. If you make your face all one colour, it just doesn't look right. Whether you're prone to redness or not, a little blush will light up your face and give it structure. We never fail to delight in the way it makes us look immediately better when we apply it in the morning.

Blush brushes

Brushes and the choice not to use them at all are always a matter of personal preference. Use what you want and when but remember, the tools you choose should be relative to the product you're using. The same brushes generally won't work for creams, gels and powders.

Keep in mind the finish you want and how much control you want to have over exactly where the product goes on the face – this will help you to choose the perfect tool for the job.

Powders work best with a fluffy brush. They need to be softly dispersed across the skin in a way that builds up light layers. Fingers, sponges and flat brushes apply powder patch-ily – it will be heavy and opaque in places, and thin or non-existent in others. Applied this way, it is also impossible to blend, so if you're a powder-blush addict, you'll need a fluffy brush, and there are loads of options.

If you are an experienced lover of blush, then a classic fluffy large(ish) blush brush is perfect. It will sweep powder gently across the apple of your cheek. You'll have slightly less control as the brush-head is larger, but the application will be quick.

If you're less experienced or prefer more control, a smaller or more pointed brush is better. The Suqqu Cheek Brush is a small but very effective little blush brush that has the same fluffy texture as a standard blush brush, but allows you to work over a smaller surface area to create exactly the effect you want.

The Real Techniques Blush Brush is large, like a standard brush, but has a tapered tip. The tip picks up the product and the bristles around it

blend the product in. This is a lovely option – you can use just the tip of the brush for precise blush or highlighter application or you can tilt the brush on its side and powder the whole face in an instant.

For cream blushes, brushes can fall short. The Nars Wet/Dry Blush Brush is tightly packed but very soft, and though it's great for powder products, it picks up and distributes creams like no other brush.

Mac's 130 Short Duo Fibre Brush is another slightly stubby brush that has a firm texture creams respond really well to. Apply your cream blush with a dabbing motion, rather than dragging it across the skin, and you'll find that it doesn't displace your foundation.

Beauty tip: Wash your brushes

You need to wash your make-up brushes. Yes, we know that it's a soul-destroyingly tedious and repetitive task, but it has to be done. There's literally no point in sticking to a care-fully considered skincare routine and then smearing age-old bacteria from filthy sponges and brushes all over your face. As your granny used to say, they're 'lighting with the dirt'.

Most people are pretty slack about brush hygiene. When we see women's make-up brushes, we sometimes wonder that the poor things haven't dragged their own crud-caked bristles to the sink in protest. You need to wash them once a week, and that's not negotiable. If you do this regularly, you'll become more aware of how matted and unpleasant brushes you use daily start to look (and smell) even after a week. If you can stretch to it, washing twice weekly wouldn't hurt.

The level of bacteria that builds up in brushes is obscene. And if that isn't enough motivation to encourage more frequent washing, when they become clogged with old product, they don't work well. A fluffy foundation brush clogged up with nasty old foundation will streak and your make-up won't look as good. A make-up artist has to wash his or her brushes after every use – just imagine how reluctant you'd be to allow them to use brushes on your face that had been unwashed for a week. Remember, the longer you leave between washes, the bigger the job it will be, so it really does minimise the workload to wash them frequently.

What you want to wash them with is up to you. There are specific brush cleansers, but who can really be bothered to pay what they cost? They aren't technically any better than anything else. Someone who is constantly washing brushes may want to use a super-gentle brush cleanser to ensure that the life expectancy of the bristles isn't compromised, but if you're a once- or twice-weekly washer, there's no need to worry or spend money on special brush cleansers.

A touch of shampoo or washing-up liquid with a small drop of olive oil added will do nicely. The olive oil will moisturise the bristles, acting like a conditioner, so that washing doesn't dry them out. Wet the brush under a tepid tap and blob some cleanser and a drop of the olive oil on the palm of your hand. Sweep the brush around your palm to make a lather, then rinse. Don't mash the bristles or tug at them: you paid for the brush and treating it gently will ensure a long lifespan. Synthetic brushes are easier to wash than natural-fibre ones because they absorb less product and tend to rinse more easily.

Repeat this process until the water runs clear through the bristles, then give them a gentle little squeeze to drain out the excess and leave them to dry. Everyone has their own theory about how you should leave brushes to dry. Some people leave theirs on a surface leaning against a wall so that the brushes are standing on their bristles. This keeps water out of the glue that bonds the bristles to the handle, but it also warps the bristles and damages their shape (along with their ability to do their job), so it isn't the best method. Never leave them vertically with the bristles facing up because the water seeps back through the bristles and sits in the glue, which will eventually cause the bond to degrade and the bristles to fall out.

The best way is to leave your brushes placed horizontally, angled a little bit forward. Prop the end of the brush on a book, and leave the bristles just barely poking over the edge of the kitchen worktop or other surface to ensure they dry back into their original shape. This protects both the bristles and the glue and it'll keep your brushes in great condition so they can serve you faithfully for years.

A touch of shampoo or washing-up liquid with a small drop of olive oil added will do nicely. The olive oil will moisturise the bristles, acting like a conditioner, so that washing doesn't dry them out.

Beauty tutorial: Applying cream blush

For a sweet, fresh-faced look, apply cream blush just to the apple of your cheek. This is the pillowy part of your cheek that forms when you grin into the mirror.

For a more sculpted, grown up look, focus the blush a little higher up towards the cheekbones.

Apply a little first, building up slowly. It's easy to add more, but hard to scale back once you've applied too much. Dab the blush into your cheek and blend the edges away with a clean finger. Be very gentle so that you don't redden your skin or pull the foundation away from underneath.

Do one side and have a look in the mirror. The side of the face with blush should look more sculpted. The made-up cheekbone should look higher and the face should look generally perkier and less flat than it did before.

Cream blush

There are lots of different formulations of blush, but the two standard kinds are cream and powder. With a cream, you'll generally get a dewier finish which gives the skin some glow and catches the light pleasingly. That is unless it's a cream-to-powder formula, in which case it will set matte – so watch out for that.

Generally, the older a woman is, the less matte finishes flatter the skin (of course, eyes are an exception). As we age, the skin naturally loses tautness and lustre, so products that reflect light give it new life. Matte formulations absorb light so they tend to look flat and quite drab, particularly on more mature skin.

When applying cream blush, always do it after foundation but before powder. The skin should be a little tacky when you apply a cream or gel blush to it. Cream and gel formulations applied over powder will clog and look mottled and uneven, more bowl of porridge than peaches and cream. You can use fingers or a brush, whichever you feel more comfortable with, but it's quite nice to apply cream blush with your fingers – it gives you ultimate control over what is going where and blends the product into the skin for a seamless finish.

If you find that applying cream blush is moving your foundation around too much, then you have one of three problems. Either you're wearing too much foundation (remember that concealer, rather than foundation, is designed to cover blemishes), you haven't buffed the foundation into the skin well enough, so your technique needs work, or you're using overly oily or emollient skincare under your foundation. Rather than dragging the blush across the skin on your finger, tap it onto the cheeks. This will leave your foundation in place and prevent streaking.

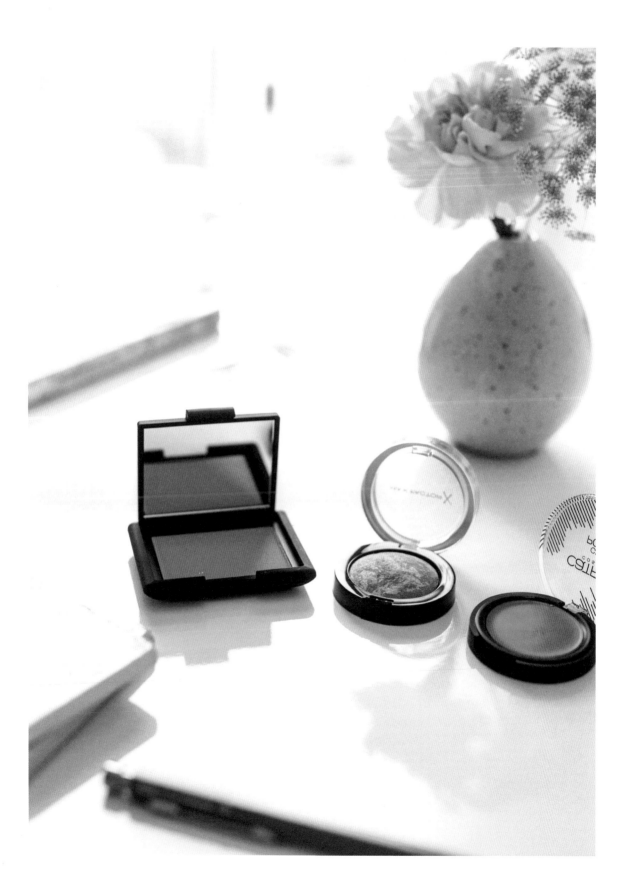

THE BEST CREAM BLUSHES

Dewy skin works beautifully on anyone, though it lasts best on drier skins. Sheerer, moister and more light-reflective formulations are much more forgiving on more mature or drier skins.

Applying powder over a dewy foundation can ruin the look, and the same goes for powder blush. Applying powder blush to an unpowdered, dewy base causes the blush to catch and sit in patches on the cheeks. This is why cream blush is a better option for drier skin or skin that you want to breathe a bit of life into. It also looks great and gives the cheeks a radiant glow, without glitter, that no powder blush can mimic. There's really no better lazy option, particularly if you're in a rush – cream blush looks great applied with fingers and can be patted on in a few seconds, so you can leave make-up brushes in the drawer and rush out the door.

Though Chanel is known for its classic powder products, they also do creams really well. Le Blush Crème de Chanel is an oil-free blush and comes in a beautiful compact. It dries down to a satin-matte finish so it has staying power without looking flat or dated. This is a feel-good, luxury buy, but the lasting power and opacity of the blush speak for themselves.

You'll use this until it's gone, and then you'll want another one.

For a sheer cream product, Burberry Beauty Fresh Glow Blush is a gorgeous option. The creamy formulation goes on smoothly, blends very easily and comes in an exciting shade range. Apply with fingers over a dewy foundation for a natural-looking flush of colour.

Mac Cremeblend Blush comes in five shades, all of which are pink-based, including brown and peachy pinks for those with sallower skin tones. Highly pigmented and setting to a dewy finish rather than the matte Chanel finish, this blush is very easy to blend. Tap it onto the apples of your cheeks with fingers for a lovely natural finish that wakes up the face.

There was a lot of excitement when Bourjois released a cream version of their iconic Little Round Pot Blush, their Little Round Pot Cream Blush, and it hasn't disappointed. Like the Chanel version, this is a cream-to-powder formula that dries quite matte and stay put all day. The formulation feels really expensive and looks brilliant on the skin. For a budget product, that's hard to top.

Now that'll put a bit of colour in your cheeks.

There's really no better lazy option – cream blush looks great applied with fingers and can be patted on in a few seconds, so you can leave make-up brushes in the drawer and rush out the door.

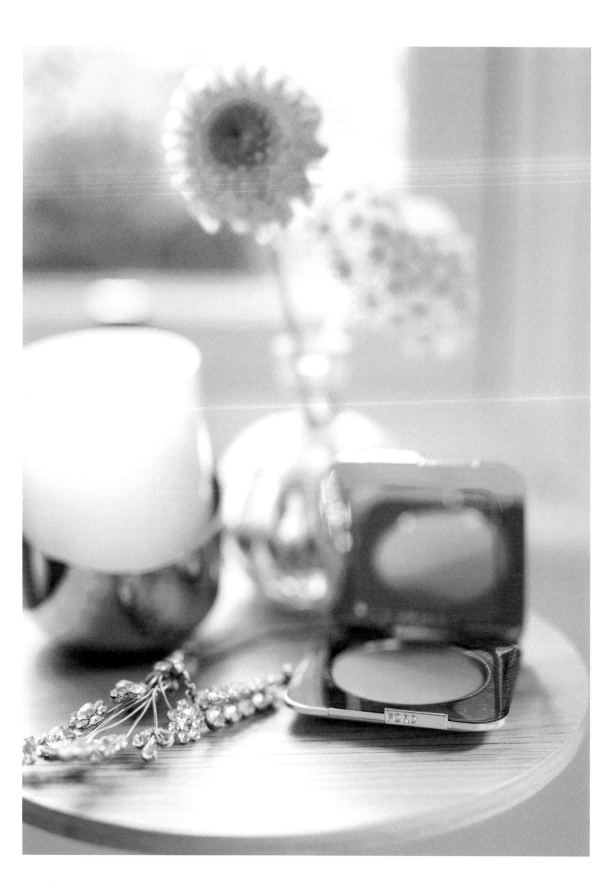

Powder blush

Powders are more traditional than creams, but no more challenging to apply. The more finely milled the powder you're using, the better the application will be. Powder blush is best applied over matte foundations or lightly-powdered foundation, but it doesn't always necessarily have a matte finish. A great powder blush won't ever leave skin flat and dull-looking. Some classic powders, like Nars Orgasm, look positively glossy on the skin. It's just a matter of buffing the powder.

You'll need a good fluffy blush brush or any brush that you've found that suits your needs. Since matte is by definition flatter in finish than cream, you can go with either a traditional matte formulation or one which is shot through with iridescent particles. The iridescent particles mimic the radiance of a creamy finish, but have more lasting power because they set on the skin and don't budge. Moist formulations are always more volatile.

The iridiscent particles in powder blush mimic the radiance of a creamy finish but have more lasting power.

Beauty tutorial: Applying powder blush

If you're using anything other than a matte foundation, powder the cheeks very lightly before applying your blush. If you don't, the powder will catch on the damp surface of the skin and you'll end up with a claggy, uneven finish just as you would when applying cream over powder. Always remember: powder over powder, cream over cream.

After powdering the cheeks lightly, swirl your clean brush in your chosen blush, then knock the excess off the brush against your wrist. You should always start light and build up to the amount you want. This creates a more natural-looking make-up, and several thin layers will last longer than one heavy blob of product. The principle of several thin layers applies to every other product in your make-up bag as well. Build up slowly – you can always add more, but it's difficult to take off excess once you've applied too much.

For a youthful, fresh-faced look, apply your blush to the apple of your cheek (the pleasingly pudgy bit that protrudes when you smile). For a more sculpted look, take it from the apple back along the cheekbone towards your hairline. Alternatively, you can buff it along your cheekbones.

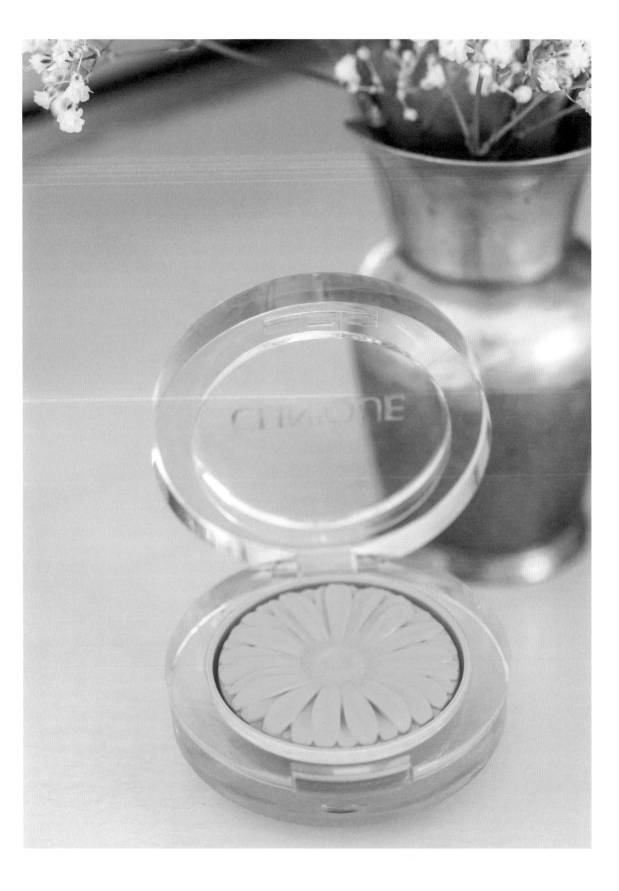

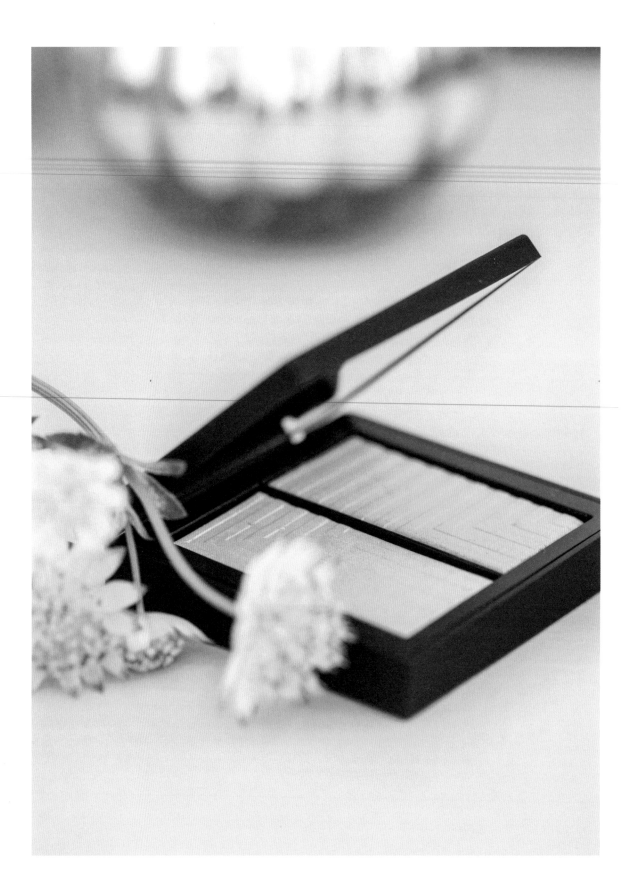

THE BEST POWDER BLUSHES

Max Factor Creme Puff Blush is a handy pocket-sized powder blush that could pass for a far more expensive product from Hourglass. Swirl a clean fluffy brush through it and dust it onto the apples of your cheeks for a wide-awake, fresh-faced look.

Nars do blush like no one else. Their cult blush, Orgasm, is a worldwide bestseller. Their formulations are buttery despite the fact that they're powders and Nars being Nars, the blushes are never one-dimensional. They always feature something interesting that makes them different, like an iridescent effect, a shocking hue or an unexpected level of pigmentation that transforms a make-up look.

For a matte finish that doesn't come in a powder formulation, Clinique Cheek Pop Blush is a brilliant option. These cute little blushes are embossed in the shape of a flower and can be applied with fingers or a brush as they have a cream-to-powder formula. They look like cream, but they apply like powder. If you like the control of applying products with your fingers but would rather not opt for a traditional powder, this lovely packs serious pigment punch and looks beautiful on the skin.

Charlotte Tilbury's Cheek to Chic Blusher is a revelation. One shade surrounded by a band of another, the glorious formulation sits on the skin perfectly. Use one shade, or the other, or both in tandem to create a tailor-made flush that reflects your mood.

Mac Mineralize Blush is a classic. It leaves an iridescence on the skin that catches the light and looks spectacular, particularly at night. It also looks wonderfully interesting in your make-up bag. Each shade is unique.

Swirl a clean fluffy brush through powder blush and dust it onto the apples of your cheeks for a wide- awake, fresh-faced look.

CHAPTER 14

· BRONZER AND HIGHLIGHTER ·

Bronzer and highlighter have been around forever, but their evolution in make-up has been fascinating. Make-up is an art form that relies on light and shadow, and bronzer and highlighter are products that create these. These products enhance and mimic natural definition in the face. Like blush, they restore the life and structure that foundation and concealer blot out, and they can be used to define and highlight particular features, ensuring that the best parts of your face steal focus.

Highlighters tend to be pretty straightforward: they generally come in liquid, cream or powder formulations and are applied to the high-points of the face to catch where the light naturally hits.

Bronzer is slightly more complex. It's available in liquid, gel, cream and powder formulations and it's often used incorrectly. Bronzer creates that pretty hue the sun gives to skin naturally after a day on the beach. The parts of the face where the sun hits – across the nose, top of the forehead and along the cheekbones – catch the sun and become a little bit darker than the rest of the face. By applying bronzer to these areas, you mimic the effect of the sun.

Beauty decoded: Contouring

Contouring was never intended as an everyday make-up skill. It's a drag and theatre make-up technique, designed to look great in certain lighting and from a distance. Contouring is illusion make-up and that sort of make-up doesn't stretch to the fluorescent lighting of your office or the stark October daylight of your kitchen.

Restructuring the face without prosthetics isn't possible. Contouring can look astonishingly good in the right lighting, but it isn't particularly convincing in real life and it definitely isn't something you need to do on a daily basis. Applying three or four different foundation shades and then blending them out with a sponge for forty minutes isn't enhancing your natural face; it's obliterating it. It's just not something that you can do every morning – you'll quickly start to feel you need to contour every day, because you'll look different without it. The moment make-up becomes something we need, it starts to feel oppressive and like a burden. That's when we know our relationship with it isn't a healthy one.

If you like the idea of trying out contouring, start by blending a small amount of foundation that's two shades darker than your skin tone underneath your cheekbones and along your hairline and make sure to blend furiously. Bad contouring looks like you've had an unfortunate run-in with orange spray paint, so proceed carefully. Remember, the darker your natural skin tone, the more contour you can get away with.

You can use anything to contour with – concealer, foundation, a neutral blush, or dedicated contour products. For dark skin tones, a very dark foundation that complements your skin works brilliantly. Paler people need to be more careful. Orangey-bronze isn't a colour that pale people tend to go, even when exposed to the sun, so stick with very subtle, almost pink-hued bronzers to mimic a soft tan. Bobbi Brown Illuminating Bronzing Powder in Antigua and NYX Taupe Powder Blush are great contouring blushes.

If you're using a cream contour product like Mac Cream Colour Base or the super-convenient Clinique Chubby Stick Sculpting Contour, rub your contour product onto the area of your palm just under your thumb. This part of the hand is the perfect size and shape to press product along the hollow of the cheekbone. Blend the edges with a clean fluffy brush for a seamless shadow.

If you like the idea of trying out contouring, start by blending a small amount of foundation that's two shades darker than your skin tone underneath your cheekbones and along your hairline and make sure to blend furiously.

Beauty decoded: Top of the cheekbones

Top of the cheekbones: The area below the temple which juts out slightly, catching the light. This is where you should apply highlighter.

Beauty decoded: Hollow of the cheekbones

Hollow of the cheekbones: Take your thumb and press gently into the cheek near the ear. The hollow you feel there is the area under-neath the cheekbone. This is where you should apply your contour products to enhance structure.

Applying bronzer and highlighter

BRONZER

If you're using bronzer under your cheekbones to define them, you should choose a matte bronzer. Anything with shimmer or light reflection will catch the light and make your features look as though they have been pushed forward.

To create realistic shadow that looks like a recess in bone structure, you need a true matte texture applied to the natural hollow in your cheek. Press your thumb into the cheek area just in front of the ear to find the hollow.

Powder bronzers should always be applied with a fluffy brush, while cream and gel formulations apply well with either a soft fluffy brush or fingers.

You can also use bronzer to mimic the effects of the sun on the skin, which is different from contouring. Bronzer should, when applied well, look like a tan. To get that lovely tanned effect, use it over a foundation that matches your skin and rely on your bronzer to add bronze hues. Using a soft fluffy brush, sweep it across the forehead and nose and wherever else the sun has a tendency to catch your face when you tan.

HIGHLIGHTER

To add extra dimension to your face and enhance your cheek-bones, apply highlighter or strobe cream along the top of cheekbones, down the centre of the nose, and across the cupid's bow.

Powder formulations should be applied with a fluffy brush, while fingers work best for cream and liquid textures.

You can also use bronzer to mimic the effects of the sun on the skin. Bronzer should, when applied well, look like a tan.

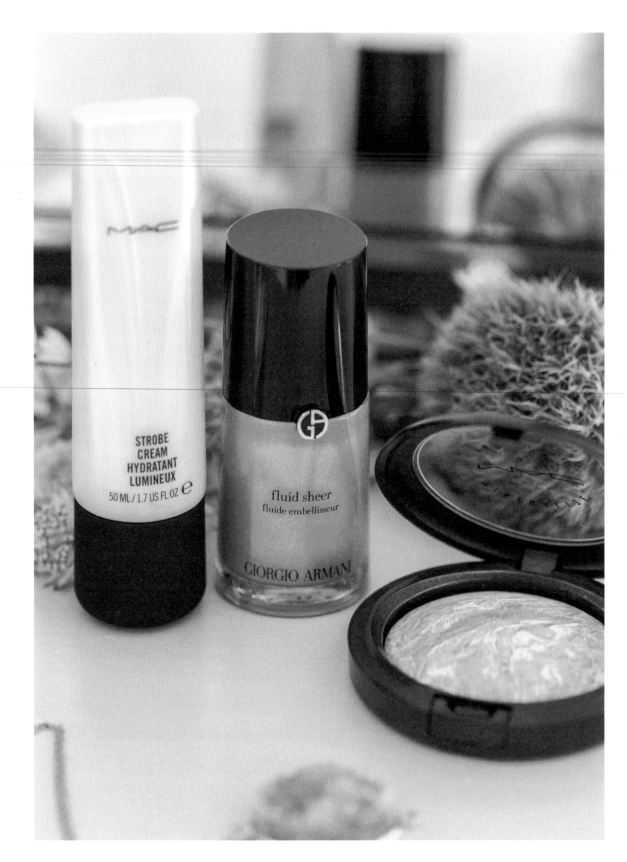

The best bronzer and highlighters

BRONZER

When it comes to bronzing, brown tones will look alien on fair skin. Natural shadows on pale people are colder in hue, tending towards grey rather than brown, so a lot of standard bronzing products on the market just don't work.

If you're pale-skinned, try Benefit Hoola, which has cooler undertones that look more natural on pale skin (though go easy or you'll look like you have dirt on your face). Nars Bronzing Powder in Laguna is also a great bronzer.

Estée Lauder Bronze Goddess All-Over Illuminator is a chunky warm-toned stick that will enable you to swipe targeted colour over cheekbones, collarbones and just about anywhere you would like to add a hint of heat. Slightly shimmering and blendable, it is nice used over lips and eyelids too.

No set of bronzing picks would be complete without a sumptuous luxury bronzer like Tom Ford's Gold Dust Bronzing Powder, a brilliant bronze that will see you through the whole bronzing season and probably the following one too. In its chic white glossy compact complete with giant mirror, this bronzer and its subtle shimmer will do you proud.

When it comes to bronzing, brown tones will look alien on fair skin. Natural shadows on pale people are colder in hue, tending towards grey rather than brown, so a lot of standard bronzing products on the market just don't work.

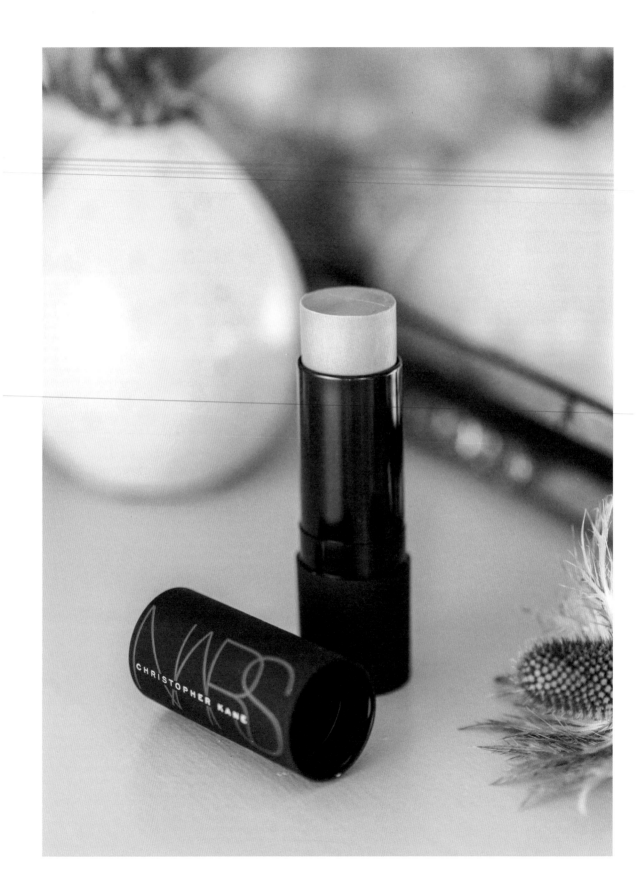

HIGHLIGHTER

The formulation of highlighter that you choose is really a matter of preference – whether you opt for a cream or a powder, the aim is silky texture and sheer glossiness.

Nars Multiple in Copacabana is a divine silver pearl cream that brings fair skin entirely to life. Dab it along the high-points of the face with an obliging finger.

A more liquid formulation like Boots Botanics All Bright Radiance Balm, Mac Strobe Cream or Charlotte Tilbury Wonder Glow can be mixed in with foundation for an all-over glow or applied where the light hits with your fingers or a brush.

With a quality powder formulation – Mac Mineralize Skinfinish in Soft & Gentle is legendary as DIY candlelit skin – the more you buff it in with a fluffy brush, the more intensely glossy it will look. Wear a little to give skin a day-time lift or a lot for an eye-catching evening look.

A cream-to-powder formula like Essence Soo Glow! Cream to Powder Highlighter is another, more affordable option for glossy, highlighted skin. It also makes a fantastic eyeshadow. We don't like limiting products to one use. Experimenting is what makes make-up fun.

We don't like limiting products to one use.
Experimenting is what makes make-up fun.

CHAPTER 15

· EYESHADOW ·

rish women are completely obsessed with that elusive beast, the smoky eye. We can't get enough of it in all its variations, from soft beige day-time versions to the full-on black blended variety. The key to a great smoky eye is blending technique with an excellent brush and two to three complimentary shades.

To begin with, get yourself four eyeshadow shades. You may want more, and you should definitely spoil yourself if you do, but you can achieve most make-up looks with a palette of four neutral shades, from beige to deep brown or black.

Opt for a quad that contains different finishes – you'll need a pale matte shade, a satin (for subtle sheen), something softly metallic like a gold or champagne shade for when you're feeling adventurous and a deep matte shade for adding depth to the eye.

Cream shadows are fantastic bases for powder shadows so try to choose a neutral cream shadow close to the shade of your natural lid to ensure that you actually get your money's worth from it.

Choosing your eyeshadow shades

Mac is the iconic brand for eyeshadow in Ireland. Their enormous range of colours and textures ensures that they will have whatever you want. All shades can be bought individually, so you don't have to buy a palette and watch several shades go to waste. You'll probably find yourself repurchasing neutral shades like Vanilla and Quarry again and again and shades you might never have considered may become your favourites. Mac Orange, which is literally a matte electric orange, is astonishing. A touch of it run through the crease of a brown-based eye make-up will bring warmth and make any eye colour pop. It looks terrifying in the pan, but small, non-obvious touches like this are what give make-up that special-looking edge.

For a shadow palette worth investing in, you don't need to look further than Dior. Their colour combinations are intelligent and beautiful, and tend to be wearable rather than overly ambitious. New limited edition palettes are released with each season's collection, so it's worth heading into a counter to see what's available.

YSL is another luxury brand that offers divine individuals shadows, while more affordable brands like Bourjois and Wet n Wild also offer lovely individuals at very competitive prices. To go all-out, opt for Urban Decay's Naked or Naked Smoky palettes.

Metallic cream shadows are more versatile than they may at first appear. As a base to layer powders on top of, they give an eye an interesting look and applied on top of a base of black eyeliner, they look stunningly glossy and exotic. A great metallic shadow can take eye make-up from day to evening in moments.

Bobbi Brown Metallic Long-Wear Cream Shadow (Goldstone is incredibly rich and autumnal) and Maybelline Colour Tattoo 24hr Eyeshadow both bring life to any make-up bag. Lancôme Colour Design Infinité 24H Eye Shadows come in rich jewel tones with a metallic finish. Chanel Illusion D'Ombre Eyeshadows are available in some more classic shades, and Rimmel Scandaleyes Eye Shadow Sticks leave a high shine, glossy finish.

Metallic cream shadows are more versatile than they may at first appear. A great metallic shadow can take eye make-up from day to evening in moments.

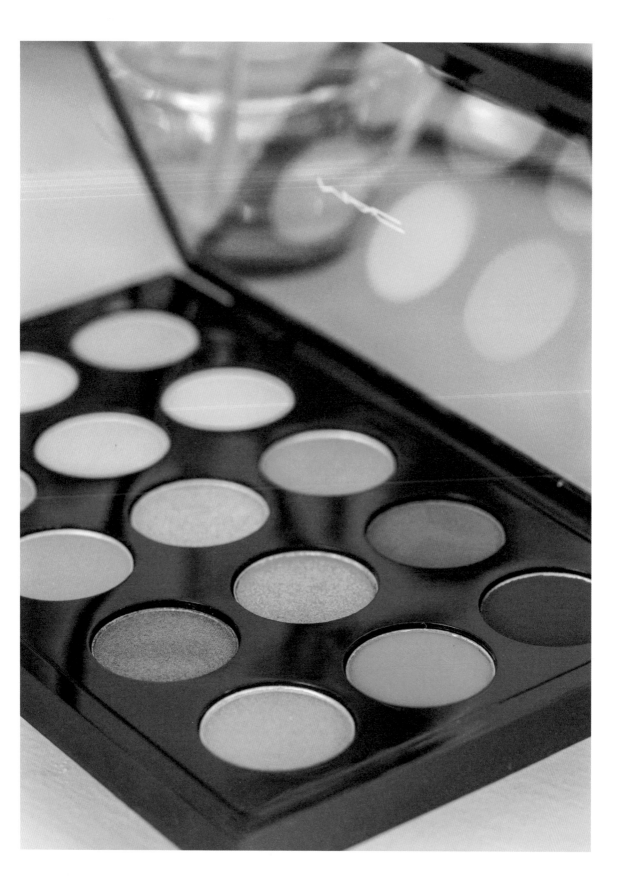

Make sure to shop around. Some brands make magnetic palettes, so that you can insert your shadows regardless of their size or brand, which is really handy.

Beauty tip: Customise your own eyeshadow palette

Loose pigment shadows that come in large pots are lovely but they make a mess, are more expensive and are harder to travel with. Instead, you should buy an empty palette to fill yourself.

Palettes from Mac come in lots of size options, from dinky little ones with space for two shadows all the way up to the big fifteen-shadow one. Inglot's Freedom System allows you to customise a palette with a range of finishes and even products – you can build a whole face of products in one palette. Urban Decay, one of the most colourful and daringly fun brands, allows you to customise an eyeshadow palette of four shades.

Make sure to shop around. Some brands make magnetic palettes, so that you can insert your shadows regardless of their size or brand, which is really handy.

To start, four shades is perfect. Think of the shades you most like and tend to wear and go for a range within that colour family, but opt for a combination of textures. A matte nude is perfect for your base colour (over primer if you want to really make an effort) applied all over the lid. Next, a slightly deeper shade, such as a taupe colour, to run through the crease (the place where your lid folds when you open your eye). Then a deeper shade – maybe a chocolate brown – to run over the outer third of the eye and through the crease. Finally, add a glitter or metallic shade to pop in the centre of the lid to catch the light and you have yourself one hell of a starter eyeshadow palette.

For a subtler day look, use just the two lighter shades; for a deeper night look, use the two darker. With four great eyeshadows, you can conquer the world.*

*of eyeshadow

Beauty decoded: Crease

Crease: The part of the eye where the lid meets the eye socket, which literally creases when your eye is open.

Eye primer

Eye primer is great product for when you need an eye look to last. It's not necessary every day, but for special occasions, it guarantees vibrancy and staying power for your eye make-up look. If you're looking to create a smoky eye using several shades of powder shadow or if your lids have a tendency to be oily, crease or move eyeshadow, applying eye primer will provide products applied after it with something to grip. Urban Decay Eyeshadow Primer Potion is a classic and comes in several shades; the shade Sin is a nice substitute for a nude cream shadow.

When you're applying lots of powder shadows (or a lot of one powder shadow), whether they're loose or pressed, they need something to grip onto so that you'll get less shadow falling down onto your cheeks.

Primers also bring out the pigment of your eyeshadow as the slightly damp surface provided by the primer intensifies the finish of your eyeshadow, making metallics look more vivid and colours look more opaque. Nars Smudge-Proof Eyeshadow Base is excellent for grip, while YSL's Couture Eye Primer is on the creamier side.

Unfortunately, eye primer seems to be one of those products that doesn't translate well to the more affordable brands. We haven't encountered and affordable eye primer to rival Urban Decay or Nars although Benefit does make good mid-range versions.

If you're not in the mood to use a primer, a cream shadow or eyeliner buffed over the lid will also make a very effective base for powder shadows, or look great all on its own. You can pop this on with a flat eyeshadow brush, or the lazy (and entirely effective) way with a finger. Try to use your ring finger because it's the weakest one and minimises the chances of accidentally jabbing yourself in the eye. It's nothing to be ashamed of. We've all done it.

Applying eye primer will provide products applied after it with something to grip.

Eyeshadow brushes

The variety of eye brushes available is dizzying, and you don't need most of them. When buying brushes, spend your money on those that do something fingers can't do. Fingers are the best thing for applying cream and gel eye products, but they can't apply powders well so a flat eyeshadow brush is essential for evenly distributing powders across the lid.

Blending is what makes eye make-up look smoky. You should never look at someone's face and be able to pinpoint the place where their eyeshadow ends. It should gradually disappear into nothingness, like a puff of smoke. Only a good blending brush can do this, and you'll use this more than any other brush in your collection. The Mac 217 Blending Brush is an unbeatable eyeshadow blending brush, while Real Techniques brushes offer brilliant quality at an affordable price.

Complete eye make-up needs eyeliner, and softening or buffing out liner is easiest with a soft pencil brush. Sharp bristles are a sign of a poor-quality brush and your eyes deserve better, so invest that bit more in a good brush if possible or use a good old-fashioned cotton bud.

With proper care, good brushes will last for years. They're worth investing in if you can.

Beauty tutorial: Blending technique for eyes

Many women are pushed to the brink of despair by the prospect of eyeshadow blending. They've tried over and over again, but just can't seem to get that soft blended edge without losing all definition or ending up with a blurry, brownish effect after two eyeshadows merge into a blob that looks like two slugs living on your eyelids.

Smoky eyes are one of the few make-up looks that can only be achieved with brushes, so it's important to get the right ones. Once you feel confident that you have the right tools, don't underestimate the importance of movement. The way you hold and move the brushes has just as much influence over the final effect as your choice of brush, so make like a ballerina with light, delicate but quick movements as you sweep the brush over your eyelids.

Take a clean fluffy blending brush – essential for a smoky eye – in your hand and blend around your eye just to observe how your hand moves. Everyone uses a brush differently but if you're nervous or inexperienced, you'll probably tend to hold the brush almost at the very tip, where the bristles emerge, which will automatically cause you to apply more force and make it difficult to blend. There is also a tendency to apply too much eyeshadow with this method.

Take a moment, relax, and hold the brush half way down the handle. It may feel strange to do this at first and as though you don't have control, but just try blending this way. You'll notice the difference in pressure against your skin. Try holding the brush at the very back of the handle for the least possible pressure on the brush and watch the effect that blending this way creates.

Powder shadows respond best to a blending technique that applies very little pressure. This will mean you'll have to take your time. It's a matter of sticking with it until a globby mess transforms into a smoky wonder. Keep at it and it will happen – you can always correct any errors with a touch of concealer. Make-up artists make mistakes all the time. The skill is in being able to fix them rather than never making them in the first place, so never beat yourself up if you go awry.

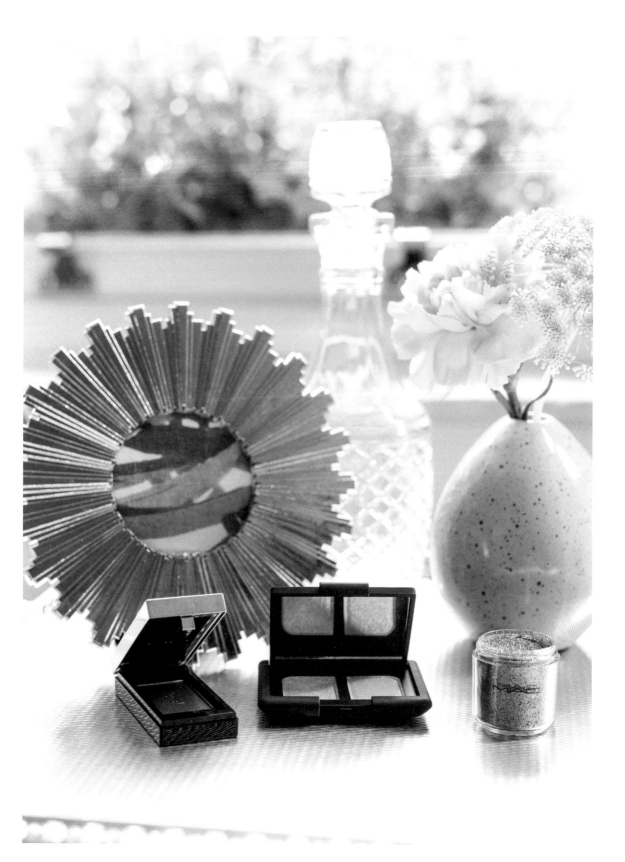

The perfect smoky eye

A smoky eye is everyone's go-to special occasion and evening make-up look. When we're out and about or in a coffee shop, we like to spend our time perving on other peoples' make-up (you know you do it too) and we regularly spy seriously good smoky eyes, from subtle daytime looks to evening eyes full of oomph. They all have one thing in common – they've taken ages and a lot of products (and sometimes a make-up artist) to achieve.

Having your make-up professionally done is a lovely option, and it's definitely one way to get the smoky eye you desire. It isn't the only way though, and can be a bit like having a professional blow-dry. You walk out of the salon with glorious, bouncy hair, but you can't recreate the effect yourself at home, and you could fly to London for less than the cost of a blow-dry in some Dublin salons.

The same goes for professional make-up application. The cost can really add up and while it's lovely for a special occasion, it's not a practical option every time you'd like a make-up look. Teaching yourself a simple smoky eye technique will allow you to create a look you feel good in whenever you're in the mood for it.

But the term 'smoky eye' can be misleading. We all know that we like a smoky eye, but if you actually ask a make-up artist to create one for you, he or she will have a litany of questions about which type you'd like. Would you prefer a day-time smoky eye? A dramatic one? Which colours would you prefer? What shape do you like the most? And on and on and on ...

So it isn't a straightforward matter of blending black eyeshadow onto the eyelid. The smoky eye comes in many forms from very simple to scarily complicated, and not all of them will look good on any one person. Your colouring, face and eye shape all factor into choosing the smoky eye that will bring your eyes to life and compliment the rest of your make-up.

If you have a hard time achieving your ideal smoky eye, start from the bottom up. We'll help you to learn a basic smoky eye technique that is beautiful on its own, and can be built on to achieve real drama.

Beauty tutorial: Nude smoky eye tutorial

That classic Mac smoky eye that you'll see girls wearing on the Mac counter is tricky and involves four or five shades of eyeshadow, as well as liner and false lashes. On the average day, ain't nobody got time for that.

If you're heading out after work, or are just in a smoky eye mood, then here's a good option for day-time.

If your eyes are close-set, then this eye make-up look will pull them outward. It also gives longer, narrower eyes a wider, rounder look. You'll need a few shadows from nude to brown, those basic colours that most of us have knocking around our make-up bag. You don't need expensive or high-end make-up for this. Just grab anything nude you have hanging around – understated colours suit everyone.

STEP 1:

- If you're off on your way to do something exciting, then apply your favourite foundation. If you're feeling more minimal, you can just apply a touch of concealer to the centre of the face and buff it out with a fluffy brush.

- Next, fill in the brows using an angled brush and two shades of matte shadow, as outlined in the brow tutorial (page 212).

STEP 2:

- Apply a shimmering or satin nude shadow all over the lid and into the inner corner to open up the eye. Pat it all over the lid with a flat eyeshadow brush.

- Next, to add some depth in the crease of the eye (the part which folds when you open your lid), grab a warm mid-toned brown. Anything warm and not too dark will work. Blend this into and along the crease of your eye with a tapered blending brush. Take your time here, sweeping the brush over and back as well as in little circles to ensure that your shadow doesn't have any hard edges. Hold the brush towards the back of the handle to ensure that you're applying very little pressure. Blending is the key to creating professional-looking make-up.

- Numerous colours ensure that this smoky eye looks interesting close up but has a lovely depth even from a distance, so next, try something like Mac's Satin Taupe, a chocolatey iridescent shade, and blend it over the top of your base colour with the same brush.

- When you get to the outer corner of the eye with your darker shade, loop the shadow down from the crease to the lower lashline, almost in the shape of a letter 'c' around the outer edge of the eye, so that the shadow at the outer corner has a slightly rounded edge. If you'd like a more elongated eye look, pull the shadow outward at the outer corner. This method works best for close-set eyes as it pulls them apart visually.

- Keep blending to ensure a lovely wispy softness to the edges.

- Finally, grab a deep aubergine shadow. You could swap this out for a deep brown or, if you want a very strong eye, a black shadow. Focus this colour on the outer corner of the eye, blending it half way along the upper lashline and into a v-shape at the outer corner of the eyelid.

STEP 3:

- If you want to bump up the look for a night-time smoky eye, just keep adding more of the deeper colours using exactly the same method and some false lashes. You'll end up with a really intense and interesting eye look. You could even add some sparkle to the centre of the lid – this will catch the light and really make your eyes pop.

- To add more definition, smudge some black pencil liner – any you have to hand will do – half way along the upper lashline to open up the eye. Don't wing it out if you want to maintain trying a rounder shape. Blend with all your might, using a blending brush or a trusty cotton bud.

- Next, some mascara (if false lashes aren't your thing). Use something volumising to really open up the eye. Two coats minimum – no messin'.

There it is. Very simple, a great starting point for all kinds of make-up looks, and so easily tailored to your own preferences. A little more liner or eyeshadow will create a very intense eye. A bit of contouring will give you a doe-eyed, sculpted look, and some false lashes and lipstick will give you full-on glamour. It's your face – dress it however feels right.

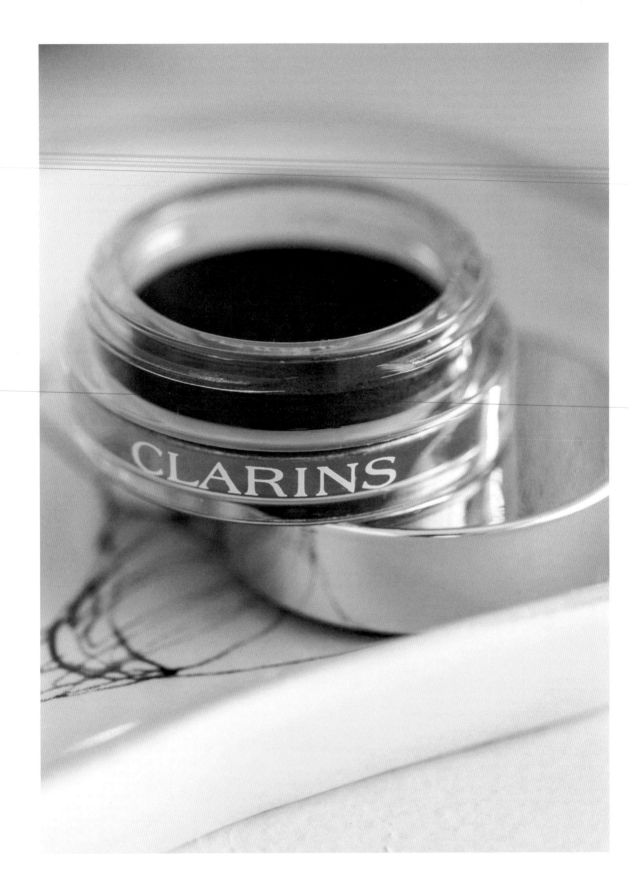

Beauty tutorial: Dramatic feline eye

This is a fresh way to modernise a classic '60s look, while maintaining all of its grungy drama. When we think of '60s make-up, it's generally a serious cat-eye, nude lips and flawless skin. The focus of the make-up was always on the eyes.

STEP 1:

- Keep your brows natural. Use a very little bit of Illamasqua Precision Brow Gel, or whatever you use, applied with an angled brush and brush your brows upward to keep them full but natural-looking.

STEP 2:

- Grab a matte beige shadow – Mac's classic neutral Brule is ideal – and pat it all over the lid with a flat eyeshadow brush.

- To achieve that dramatic '60s contour, take a matte grey colour and buff it along the crease of your eye (where it folds when open) with a fluffy brush. Wing it out past the stopping point of the eye and blend with a clean fluffy blending brush until any harsh lines disappear.

STEP 3:

- Grab your black gel liner and with a fine liner brush, draw in your flick first.

- You need to draw the flick in lower than usual as it needs to be joined seamlessly to the liner on your lower lashline later. So draw in your flick, extending it out quite far, and work backwards towards the inner corner, building your liner into a feline flick that is thinner at the inner corner but quite thick overall.

- Keep your cotton buds on hand to tidy up your flick if needed. Everyone makes mistakes; just be patient with yourself and tidy up any errors as you make them.

- When you're happy with it, take a pencil liner in black and dot it along the lower lashline. Don't worry if it looks messy – you'll be blending it next.

- With a pencil brush, blend your black liner, smudging it all along the lower lashline and joining it to the flick on your eyelid, as in the picture.

- Line your upper and lower waterlines, wiggling the liner right into the lashes to prevent any gaps.

- Apply a coat (or three) of your favourite volumising mascara, or if you're feeling brave, some false lashes.

Finish the look with some contouring and a nude lip and you're done, a '60s feline queen.

CHAPTER 16

· EYELINER ·

Eyeliner was first used in Ancient Egypt and Mesopotamia and has been around for literally thousands of years. There's a reason we still love it today and that it has endured for such a long time. The right liner and application style is better than any scalpel – you can use it to alter the shape of your eyes to suit your mood.

Laura's love affair with gel and liquid liners began in her teens. She went through the usual phase of trying different products and looks (many of which were pretty bad) before being given the gift of a pot of gel liner and a fine liner brush. Fascinated by old Hollywood actresses like Audrey Hepburn and Marilyn Monroe, along with the beauty of their groundbreaking make-up, Laura knew she'd found the look she wanted to wear. Several weeks of dogged practise ensued until her first passable cat-eye was created. She'd found her thing, and has worn a classic '50s liner almost every day since. She maintains that it transforms her rounder eyes into a slightly more almond shape and it feels incredibly chic. After years of practise, it takes just two minutes in the morning.

Depending on the mood you're in and the look you want to create, you can use liner to change your eye shape. It's the most surgical everyday make-up tool we have.

A line that is thicker towards the centre of the eye and thinner at the edges creates a rounded appearance to your eyes, as does taking liner partially along your lower lashline from the outer corner. An elaborate flick that points aggressively upward gives the illusion of pulling your eye up, creating the impression of an almond shape. A flick that points downward pulls the outer corner of the eye down and creates a sort of manga character look, while a straight long line from the inner corner over to the outer corner makes the eye look longer. For a more feline-looking eye, draw a long, straight liner flick, and fill in the lower waterline, narrowing and elongating your eyes.

Beauty decoded: Waterline

Waterline: The rim of bare area inside the eyelashes which touches the eye.

Beauty decoded: Outer third of the eyelid

Outer third of the eyelid: Imagine your eye in three sections. The outer third is the last section where it joins the temple, the area of the eyelid above where your lashes end.

The best type of eyeliner

While old-fashioned kohl liners are great, we think that a gel is the most versatile formula. You can use gel for smudging and for creating super-clean lines or just buff it all over the lid with a fluffy eye brush to create a base for powders which will work exactly like a cream shadow.

Classic smudgy kohl liners are just that – smudgy. For a worn-in, grungy make-up look, they cannot be beaten and as a base for powder eyeshadow, they're excellent. But as the day (or night) progresses, kohl will move. Generally downward, and in an unforgiving fashion.

A gel liner can be smudged like a kohl while wet but once set, it won't move. It also gives you hyper-precise clean lines, which is what's needed for a cat-eye. It has all the benefits of both kohl and liquid liner, without any of the drawbacks – although if you have hooded eyes, you may find gel liner smudges, so turn to liquid instead.

Liquid liners are every bit as good as gels for creating clean lines, but they have two shortcomings: one, you can't blend them as they just streak and look awful, making them a decided no for anything other than precise eyelining; and two, they always come in horrible packaging. With a tub of gel liner, you get to choose the type and shape of brush that you find easiest to work with. Liquid liners traditionally come in a small tube with a twist-off lid that has a brush attached and these brushes are terrible. They're too soft, the bristles are too long and they often make lining far harder than it needs to be.

Classic smudgy kohl liners are just that – smudgy. For a worn-in, grungy make-up look, they cannot be beaten and as a base for powder eyeshadow, they're excellent.

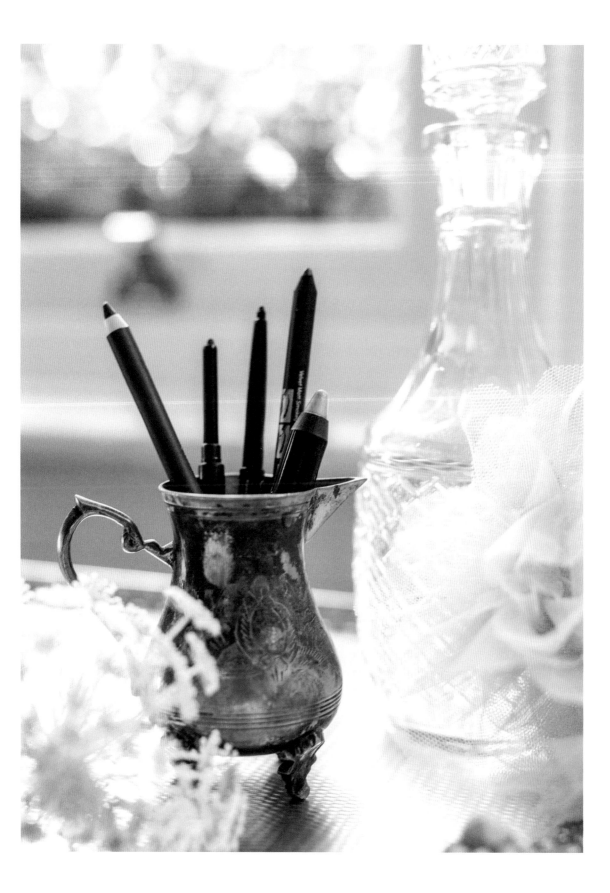

The best eyeliners

The effects you can create with eyeliner are pretty much endless. Go for a grungy smear of kohl or a clean '50s flick. Line the inner waterline to elongate the eyes or just line the outer third to widen them. If you change the colour, with a cat-eye flick in a bright blue or white, for example, you change the feel of the whole make-up. Lining eyes may seem tough but it's a skill you can improve on with practice, and it opens up endless opportunity for fun and expression with make-up.

Benefit They're Real Push Up Liner makes the task of creating a cat-eye, complete with a flick, far easier to do. The rubber applicator is gentle on the eye, especially if you're prone to accidental eye jabs. Pushing it gently along the lashline will create your line for you, eliminating most of the dirty work.

Bobbi Brown Ink Liner is a classic precision felt-tip liner. Like Charlotte Tilbury Feline Flick Quick Fine Line Shodõ Pen, it is more of a liquid than a gel, and won't blend very well, but it creates a flawlessly clean line that won't budge. If felt-tip liners aren't your cup of tea, Lancôme Artliner Eyeliner is a classic wand liquid liner available in lots of colours.

Maybelline Eye Studio Lasting Drama Gel Eyeliner may have a name that takes more time to say than the stuff takes to apply, but it is Laura's favourite. In quality, it matches higher-end equivalent gel pot liners by Bobbi Brown and Laura Mercier and the colour is black as a priest's socks. The pot makes it incredibly versatile as you can use different brushes for different effects. It is also available in a range of different colours. For

The effects you can create with eyeliner are pretty much endless. Go for a grungy smear of kohl or a clean '50s flick. Line the inner waterline to elongate the eyes or just line the outer third to widen them.

EYELINER | CHAPTER 16

*Lining eyes may seem tough but it's a skill you can
improve on with practice, and it opens up endless
opportunity for fun and expression with make-up.*

an even more affordable option that stays put, try Catrice Waterproof Gel Eye Liner.

Most pot liners have one drawback – they tend to dry out quickly. Laura Mercier Crème Eye Liner is the one exception we've found. It is on the pricey side but it won't dry out in the pot and is perfectly pigmented. The slightly wetter formula is also easier for beginners to use and it's available in a host of fun colours, not just black.

NYX Curve Eyeliner is a slightly weird, space-agey gadget that you might be a bit frightened of when you first see it. The curve is designed to fit snugly between thumb and index finger to steady the hand and create a perfect line. It is more a liquid than a gel but it either blends or creates a perfect clean line, depending on what you want. Once it sets, this stuff isn't budging.

For a traditional smudgy kohl pencil, you can't beat Mac Feline Kohl Power Eye Pencil or Elizabeth Arden Smoky Eyes Powder Pencil, which was Charlotte Tilbury's lifelong favourite for her famous cat-eye look before she developed her own Rock 'n' Kohl Eye Pencil, which creates a slightly unwieldy grunge-inspired eye with a lived-in look. Smudged underneath some powder eyeshadow, it's creamy enough to create the grip needed to hold powders in place while intensifying their colour. Don't rely on this liner for a clean '50s liner look – this is for your rock chick moments.

Beauty tutorial: How to apply eyeliner

If you're a total eyeliner novice or have a pathologically shaky hand, it's easy to think of a cat-eye as the unreachable make-up dream. Eyeliner is everyone's Holy Grail make-up technique. A perfect flick garners more compliments than any other make-up look or technique and it looks good on every kind of eye. Yes, you have to adjust the technique for certain eye shapes, and the younger you are, the thicker the line you can get away with, but if you thought you could never get away with wearing a classic eyeliner flick, think again.

Here are the tips to achieve the liner look that will always attract admiration:

STEP 1:

- If you're a total novice, start with a soft liner pencil. A gel pencil will go on most smoothly. Don't worry if you'd rather use gel or liquid liner – just draw a template of your flick initially with the pencil, and then trace over it with your chosen liner. A pencil is easier to manipulate if you're not confident with liner. Just be sure to use something that will set and dry, like a gel pencil. If you use kohl, it will be all over your eyelids and under your eyes by lunch.

- Urban Decay's 24/7 Glide-On Eye Pencil in Perversion is a gorgeously buttery gel texture that doesn't move once dry. Sharpen your pencil to a nice point (make sure not to try this with a poor-quality pencil – they can often be too sharp and damage the eye). Test the pencil on the back of your hand first to make sure that it is soft enough.

- A good gel pencil is entirely worth investing in – the higher the quality, the softer the texture and the less it will move once dry.

- When you're ready, draw a basic line along the upper lashline. Try resting your little finger on your face as you go. This provides balance and will stop your hand from shaking. Laura finds if she tries to apply a line without resting her pinky on her cheek for balance, her hand shakes and she messes up the liner completely, so don't worry if you've had this problem. The simple act of balancing your hand might just unlock the perfect liner you've always wanted.

- Start at the outer corner of the eye and work your way into the inner corner. Keep the line thin all the way along. You'll be able to refine it later. Again, if the pencil is not good quality, this will be uncomfortable and require lots of poking and retracing, so use something soft and reliable.

- The line should stop at the very end of the upper lashline – ending it sooner makes it more difficult for a beginner to create two matching flicks.

STEP 2:

- Begin extending the liner up and out into a flick.

- Imagine that the lower lashline continued up in an imaginary liner – that's the line you're following with your pencil.

- All the time, keep balancing that little finger on your cheek to keep your hand steady.

STEP 3:

- Next, take the pencil back towards the lid, creating a little triangle. This will be the flick. Take your time with this part and don't despair if you make an error. A little cotton bud or a damp tissue over the edge of your fingernail will clean up your lines in a jiffy.

- Draw the line all the way back to the inner corner, ensuring that it's thinner there than it is at the outer corner.

- If you have hooded eyes, you can absolutely still wear a flick. The problem with lining hooded eyes is that a liner that is perfect when your eyes are shut will bend when they're open. The solution? Draw your flick on with your eyes open, looking head on into a mirror. The flick should be drawn on further away from the lid at the outer corner so that it stays still even when you blink. Gel or kohl liners are not recommended for clean liner looks on hooded eyes as they can smudge. Instead, try liquid or marker styles like Shu Uemura calligraph:ink Liquid Eyeliner.

STEP 4:

- Fill in the liner and apply a liquid or pot gel over the top if you want a really clean line. The flick should be quite far out; that way it won't move when your eyes do.

If it's not perfect, don't fret. You're well on your way to mastering the cat-eye of your dreams. Remember to have patience with yourself. Lining eyes takes precision and is a skill which takes time to perfect. Keep your cotton buds handy and practice. It's easier than you think.

Remember to have patience with yourself.
Lining eyes takes precision and is a skill
which takes time to perfect.

CHAPTER 17

· MASCARA ·

Mascara has to be the most recognisable cosmetic product of them all. Everyone, regardless of gender or age, knows what it is. That's possibly because it looks pretty insane to have a spiny brush that close to your eye.

Mascara is such a big deal that, on average, an enormous two hundred brand new mascaras are released each year, meaning there are approximately two million for us to choose from. A slight exaggeration perhaps, but most makeup-wearing women will spend thousands on mascara over their lifetimes.

Mascara's importance to the cosmetics industry means that the fight for market share leads to ever more ridiculous claims and brush types – L'Oréal even employs someone whose sole job is to develop mascara brushes (they call him the 'wand wizard'), but there are few products more subject to personal preference than mascara. While some people hate that spidery, cloggy look, others love it. Some of us want subtle definition; others want false lashes in a tube. The one thing we generally agree on is that mascara should be black as a witch's *gúna* and should lengthen and thicken the lashes to our preferred degree. We'll have no insipid, greyish watery business here. We want the real deal.

Mascara has a life span of between three to five months, which might explain why we prefer not to spend too much on it. After that time, it will thicken, eventually turning to dust. More importantly, after its recommended life span, it is no longer sanitary and you risk eye infection. Fantastic lashes on a swollen, oozing eye don't really enhance it, so make sure to bite the bullet and bin your mascara if you've had it for five months or more. Nothing is worth an eye infection.

Do remember, though, that brushes can be reused. If you love a particular brush, wash it thoroughly and hang onto it to try with another mascara formula. Odds are you'll prefer the finish you get to the brush that comes with the mascara.

Applying mascara

It seems like a dangerous waste of money, but the one way to ensure perfect, clog-free mascara application is to wipe the brush thoroughly in a tissue when you remove it from the tube. Most of the mascara will be left in the tissue so if it's expensive you'll be calculating how many euros are currently clotting up in a tissue beside you, but the effect on your lashes will immediately be better. Mascara works by the same principle as all other make-up: several thin layers stay longer and look better than one quickly hefted-on blob. Two thin coats of your favourite mascara will give you lift, length and volume without any stickiness or clogging.

Since we use oil-based cleanser to take off waterproof mascara, it won't fare particularly well on someone with an oily eye area. Sweat and sebum are oil-based, and these are what cause your mascara to dissolve and move.

Look for smudge-proof mascara instead as it's more likely to stay put for longer, and minimise the problem by using an eye primer on the lid before applying mascara. Some handy smudge-proof options are NYC City Proof 24hr Waterproof Mascara (which is smudge-proof as well as waterproof) and Bobbi Brown No Smudge Mascara.

If you happen to make a mistake and get a blob of mascara on the skin around your eye, it's easily fixed. Professional make-up artists make just as many mistakes as everyone else; they just know how to fix them. Don't tackle the blob while it's wet. Leave it to dry completely, then take a dry cotton bud and lift off the dried mascara in a gentle rolling motion. Your eye make-up will remain intact and you can go about your business. Crisis averted.

Mascara works by the same principle as all other make-up: several thin layers stay longer and look better than one quickly hefted-on blob. Two thin coats of your favourite mascara will give you lift, length and volume without any stickiness or clogging.

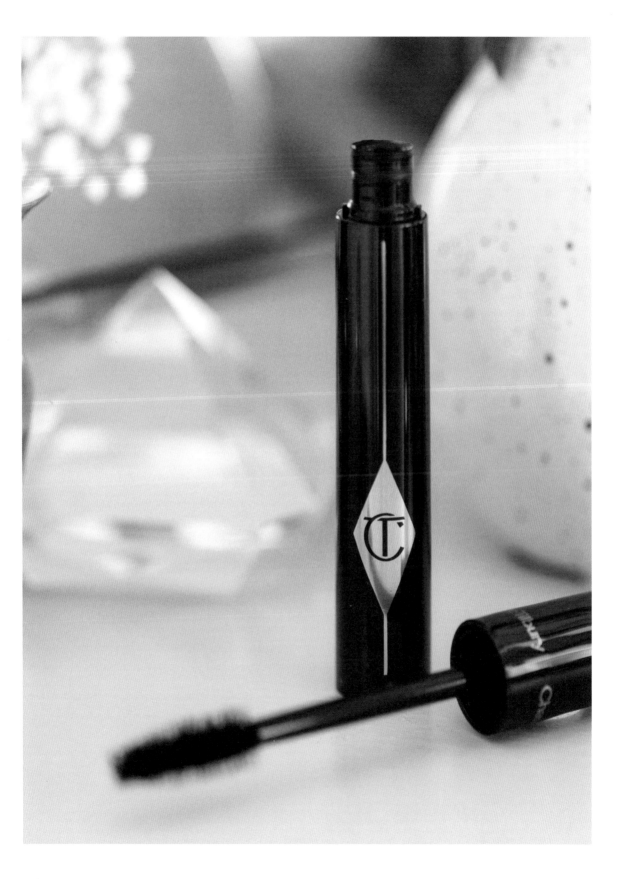

Beauty decoded: Volume Seekers

'Volume Seeker' is the special name given by the cosmetic industry to women who crave extreme lash thickening. While the average woman swipes the mascara wand five or six times over her lashes, Volume Seekers are not be satisfied with fewer than thirty or forty coats. This essentially turns lashes into a solid lump of mascara so the Volume Seekers need to separate their lashes. They do this with pins, needles, earring spikes or whatever sharp and dangerous implement is lying around. Puncturing the eyeball has been known to occur, but Volume Seekers don't worry about this inconvenience – they want volume and they don't care what it takes.

Our recommendation? Buy some false lashes instead.

The best mascaras

We loathe rubber mascara wands. We've never encountered one that works – the product clogs in them and drips thickly onto the lashes, sticking them together. They can work, but only if you wipe them almost completely clean of product before applying them. This is vastly irritating and our grannies' voices ring about 'thrift' in our heads every time we use mascara with a rubber brush.

Still, if you don't mind the wastage, some of the mascaras on the market that come with a rubber brush, such as Benefit They're Real Mascara (the bestselling mascara globally of any brand) and Lancôme Grandiose Mascara, are great.

A traditional bristled brush tends to distribute the formula better, and the thinness and flexibility of the bristles is more likely to separate individual lashes from one another than a rubber spoolie, which catches lashes in little tufts of several at a time.

If, like us, you prefer a traditional bristled mascara brush, then you can't beat YSL Luxurious Mascara For False Lash Effect. Eye-wateringly expensive for something with such a short lifespan, it is nonetheless fantastic and gives lashes an incomparable finish. The same goes for Charlotte Tilbury Full Fat Lashes and Urban Decay Perversion Mascara.

Rubber mascara wands can work, but only if you wipe them almost completely clean of product before applying them.

A traditional bristled brush tends to distribute the formula better, and the thinness and flexibility of the bristles is more likely to separate individual lashes from one another than a rubber spoolie,

Smashbox Full Exposure Mascara has a big, abundant brush that lengthens lashes beautifully, while the more affordable Maybelline Falsies Big Eyes Mascara offers two brushes in one tube so that you can customise the volume to your mood. The smaller brush catches the smaller lashes on either side of the eye without globbing the formula all over your eyelid.

For contact lens wearers with sensitive eyes trying to avoid smudges and panda eyes, Trish McEvoy Lash Curling Mascara is perfect. Though pricey, once you've tried this mascara you'll start saving every cent in order to buy it again and again. If you have mild rosacea and find some mascaras can cause irritation, this is ideal and won't cause your eyes to get itchy.

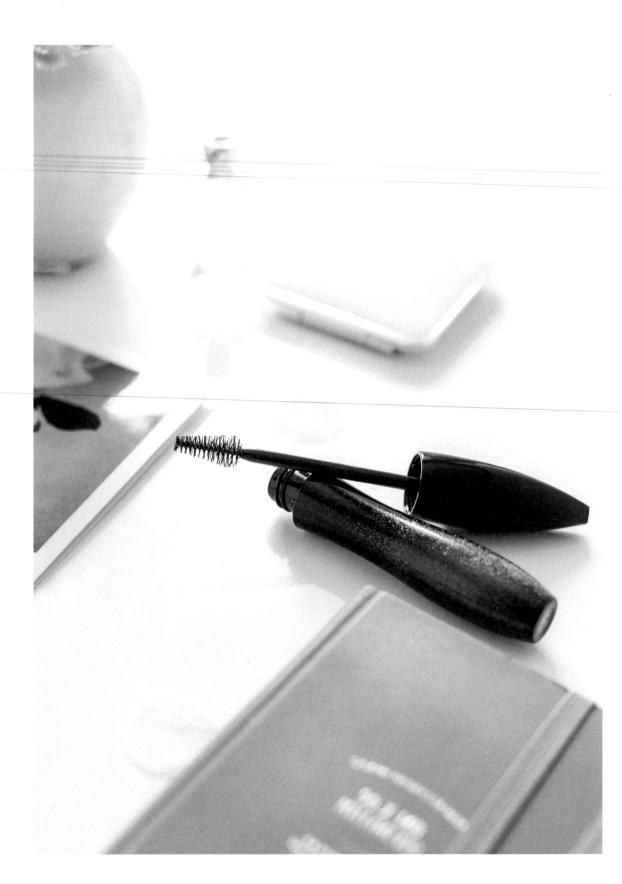

False lashes

False lashes are a great way to amp up an eye look with very little effort. They can be tricky to apply at first, but once you get the hang of it, you'll have them on in no time.

Firstly, the quality of the lashes you choose is important. Very cheap lashes look synthetic (i.e. have an obvious, plastic-looking shine to them) and have a very thick lash band. This is the strip that the false lashes are attached to. If it's very thick, it will look obvious on the eye and won't be as flexible, making the lashes far harder to apply.

If you're a lash novice, choose quality individuals – these are little tufts of lashes that are much more subtle than a classic strip lash. They're easier to apply, have no lash band that you need to conceal and most importantly, you can't feel them on the eye the way you can feel a strip of lashes. Individual lashes are also far more versatile than strips. Wear a couple on the outer corner of the eye for flutter, or wear masses of them to hugely volumise your lashes for a special occasion.

Eylure and Ardell both offer affordable, quality individual lashes. Just be aware that the long ones in a combination pack are always too long for everyone – stick to medium and short lengths, focusing the short lashes from the inner corner to the centre and the medium lashes from the centre to the outer corner. This will give you a lazy Marilyn Monroe look.

When wearing strip lashes, check if they are longer than your eye. If they are, trim them carefully. Apply a thin layer of glue to the band and wait for at least thirty seconds. Make sure to use a high-quality glue – Duo Eyelash Adhesive is the best and comes in white, which dries down to clear, and black. Then apply the centre of the false lash band to the centre of your lashline, applying it to the skin just above rather than directly onto the lashes. Next, take the edges of your false lashes, and attach them to the corners of your eye. If they don't stick, you haven't left the glue long enough before applying. Wait a few seconds, and try again.

When the lash glue is dry, it may leave a shiny residue. If it does, go over it with black liner to disguise it. When you remove your lashes, pick off the glue and put them back in the box – you should be able to wear them several times before they start to look tired.

Individual lashes are also far more versatile than strips. Wear a couple on the outer corner of the eye for flutter, or wear masses of them to hugely volumise your lashes for a special occasion.

Make-up is about light and shadow, just like any other art form. You might wear more for a selfie than you would ordinarily but the trick is to capture an image of yourself at your realistic best, so opt for nicely polished everyday make-up.

Beauty decoded: Selfie make-up

Over seventeen million selfies are uploaded to social media each week, so it seems that we're becomingly increasingly interested in our own faces. A quick Google search turns up masses of 'selfie tutorials', and while make-up for photography might involve a few more visual tricks than everyday make-up, it doesn't mean that good old-fashioned application techniques don't work just as well.

Make-up is about light and shadow, just like any other art form. You might wear more for a selfie than you would ordinarily but the trick is to capture an image of yourself at your realistic best, so opt for nicely polished everyday make-up.

With selfies, there's always the option to go full-on unrealistic by editing the bejaysus out of your photos. The emergence of photo-editing apps for selfies is, in some ways, very comforting. It allows normal women to see just how photoshopped advertising images really are. If you can use a free app to blast away lines and blemishes to the point where you barely recognise your own face, then imagine the help that celebrities have. They simply don't look the way photos imply they look.

When an untouched photograph of Beyoncé emerged last year, it caused all manner of fuss. When people saw that one of the world's most beautiful women had actual human skin with actual human imperfections, some reacted with horror (eejits) and others felt surprised that Beyoncé isn't completely perfect. But nobody is. Beyoncé is blindingly gorgeous, but it's good for people to know that perfectly airbrushed skin doesn't really exist, even for the massively wealthy, and accepting yourself as imperfect isn't a form of giving up.

Kim Kardashian confessed that she takes at least three hundred photos for every one she chooses to upload. That sort of devotion to narcissism is pretty terrifying and in real life it is simply impossible to achieve, no matter how much of a vanity smurf you are. You'd never have time to finish drying your hair or get to the post office before it closes at that rate.

Now that we know that selfies – at least the classic celebrity ones – are based pretty much entirely on lies and a fierce amount of effort, we can feel a bit better about them.

If you like the idea of a little extra help in the form of a photo-editing app that blasts away blemishes and magically eradicate lines, there are lots to choose from. PhotoWonder, Facetune and Perfect365 all airbrush you to within an inch of your life if that's what you're into, but don't become so reliant on editing apps that you stop being able to recognise the best aspects of your face – the artificial standard created by Photoshop runs that risk.

If you're concerned about selfie make-up, a great concealer is the product to cover blemishes and disguise dark circles. Clarins Instant Concealer offers coverage to disguise the most sleepless of nights and applied under foundation where needed, provides the perfect canvas for photography.

Facial definition can get lost in photographs, particularly if you're using a flash, so sweeping a matte contour product under the cheekbones – Illamasqua Cream Pigment in Hollow is especially perfect for very pale Irish complexions – helps to pull in their natural hollow and accentuate their shape. Pair this with a highlighter across the top of the cheekbones, as well as down the nose and on the cupid's bow.

Highlighter pushes any feature it is applied to outward as it catches the light. Mac Mineralize Skinfinish in Soft & Gentle is a classic choice, with a finish like powdered candlelight, and Bobbi Brown Shimmer Bricks are lovely powder highlighters that come in shades for every skin tone.

While carefully placed shine adds definition, shine in the wrong place will throw off the photograph and make your face look oily. Powder the centre of the face, particularly around the nose, if needed.

Since definition enhances your features, it would be a mistake to forget your brows. A cure-all brow kit like Brow Zings Brow Shaping Kit from Benefit contains everything you need to enhance them for a sharp but natural-looking finish.

Finally, you can't go wrong with a red lipstick. A blue-toned classic red or a hot pink whitens the teeth and gives the face the essential definition to keep it from looking flat or dull in photos. L'Oréal Color Riche in True Red is a nice affordable option.

When it comes to taking the photo, more is more. Take as many as you can, testing different lights and angles until you find the right one. Don't pull a duck face and you're 80% there already.

While carefully placed shine adds definition, shine in the wrong place will throw off the photograph and make your face look oily. Powder the centre of the face, particularly around the nose, if needed.

CHAPTER 18

· EYEBROWS ·

Most of us spent our teens ripping our brows from our faces with the same determined expression your granny has when she weeds her garden, and now we all want them back. We may not exactly crave Cara Delevingne's caterpillar brows, but a fuller and more natural look is certainly regaining popularity.

After years of emphasis on perfectly groomed brows, it's finally become acceptable to let them grow wild and free. You can give them a comb with some brow mascara, groom them to within of their lives or leave them to waggle proudly bare in the wind like a field of wheat – anything goes.

Brow shapes can be manipulated with make-up, but keep in mind that your natural shape will always look good on you so try to use your natural brow shape as your guide. If you have poker-straight brows, forcing a high arch into them won't look natural and you'll need lots of brow make-up to pull it off. If your brows have a naturally high arch, then it will be very difficult to make them look straight without plucking or piling on make-up.

Growing your brows

Growing brows back can be tremendously frustrating and slow. If you haven't been kind to them over the years, then they'll take their time to resurface, like a frightened tortoise working the courage up to pop his head out of his shell. Be patient and give it time. While you wait, look out among friends, co-workers and family – when you come across someone with great brows, ask how they achieved them.

There are several horrible stages of growing your brows out, from the dirty-looking little black dots that appear as the hairs first start to form to the straggly little feckers who decide to position themselves wherever they want.

If you haven't got much going on in the brow department, you'll just have to accept the fact that your eyebrows will grow back in the shape of the 145 bus route and hold yourself back from tweezing for a while. It can be tough to have all the scrubby undergrowth bristling out all over the place, but have patience. If you go in with a tweezers to catch that one hair that is annoying you more than any other, before you know it you'll have got it and then gone back for the rest, at which point you'll be back where you started.

Look out among friends, co-workers and family – when you come across someone with great brows, ask how they achieved them.

Tinting your brows

Tinting the brows is underrated. Don't be put off by having to take a little bit of time to do it. A professional brow tint and shape is an option, but it can be costly if you're doing it regularly. You can easily tint your own brows at home.

Colorsport 30 Day Mascara Eyelash & Brow Dye Kit comes in a great brown shade that will work well for anyone with naturally brown or black brows. If you're a natural blonde and want to lend drama and structure to your face, the brown shade is a good option. It doesn't contain any nasty red undertones, which look unnatural and odd on anyone who isn't a redhead.

Eylure Permanent Tint for Brows is another great option. It catches all the fine whitish hairs that you can't see with the naked eye to give you more brow. Tinting your brows yourself takes under ten minutes and makes an enormous difference to their size and shape. You immediately have more eyebrow to work with than you realised and it opens up the option of going without make-up on your brows.

Tinting your brows yourself takes under ten minutes and makes an enormous difference to their size and shape. You immediately have more eyebrow to work with than you realised and it opens up the option of going without make-up on your brows.

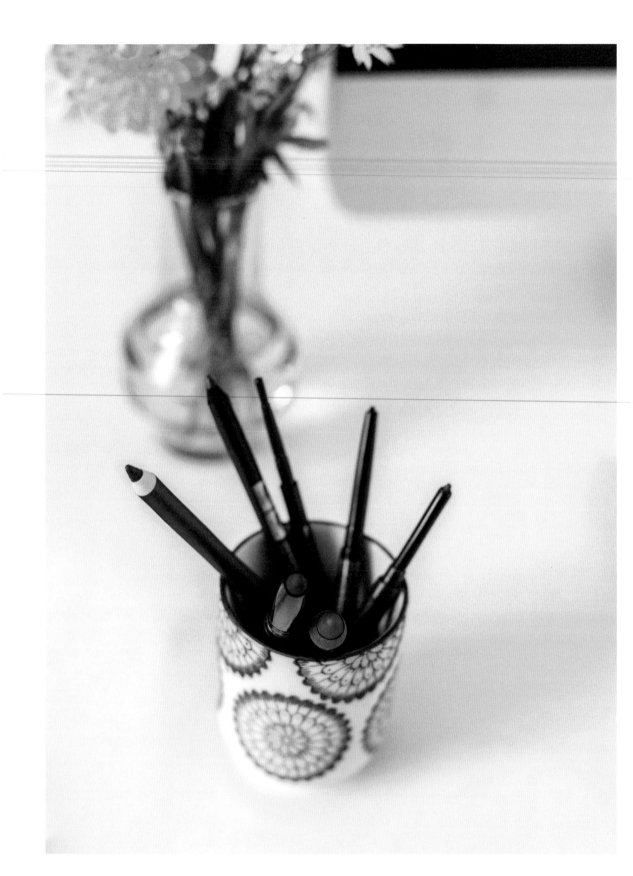

Always brush through brows with a brow comb or spoolie after applying brow pencil or it may look hard.

The best brow products

Different brow products produce different finishes. For a sculpted, full brow, opt for a gel product. Illamasqua Brow Gel applied with an angled brush cheats fullness and very clean lines. Focus the majority of the product towards the outer edge of the brow and always brush through brows with a clean mascara wand after to get rid of any harshness. The permanent-marker brow look doesn't work for anyone.

For a softer look, choose a pencil. Clarins eyebrow pencils are the perfect consistency – hard enough to draw in individual hairs, but soft enough to apply comfortably and blend. Always brush through brows with a brow comb or spoolie after applying brow pencil or it may look hard.

Affordable brow products absolutely rival their pricier counterparts. For an enhanced but natural finish, brush a brow mascara through your eyebrows. L'Oréal Brow Artist Plumper is a great choice. It adds definition and coats the finer hairs, making brows look fuller without looking like make-up or taking any effort.

If you're looking for brow brushes, Estée Lauder, Bobbi Brown and Eco Tool all do good ones. You can get good brow brushes from most brands but we recommend investing – brows are a daily staple.

For a finish that's more made-up than mascara but less 'done' than gel, opt for an old-fashioned powder. Benefit Brow Zings Brow Shaping Kit contains brow powder and a wax to set hairs in place. It comes in shades to suit every hair colour and lasts for months.

Beauty tutorial: Create a full brow

There are all sorts of fussy brow products on the market but a basic brow doesn't need them. Using two powder eyeshadows creates a softer look than pencil or gels and mimics the naturally very slightly patchy look of natural brows while providing soft fullness and definition. Using one shade will never mimic the variety of natural brows. Opt for two and you'll be shocked by the definition they provide.

Here's what you need to create a natural-looking, full brow:

- A good angled liner brush, not too stiff, not too soft: it should give just a little when you push the bristles. Try the Mac 266 Small Angle Brush.

- A brow comb or spoolie: natural hair gives a better finish than synthetic when you're brushing brows through, but there's no need to invest in an expensive brush.

- Two matte eyeshadows in your brow colour: we suggest one light and one deep brown. If you're blonde, you'll need a very light brown/dark blonde shade and a slightly darker shade. Always stick to matte finishes. Unless your hair is literally black, avoid black altogether. If you're a redhead, try two warm brown shades, one light, one deeper, rather than cooler brown shades.

Using two powder eyeshadows creates a softer look than pencil or gels and mimics the naturally very slightly patchy look of natural brows while providing soft fullness and definition.

STEP 1:

- Brush your brows through so that the hairs are lying in whatever is the natural direction of their growth. Then, using your angled brush, apply your lighter brown shade along the bottom of the brow. Take your time and create a nice neat line. Don't worry too much about precision as the powder ensures a soft finish. You can't really apply the light colour too heavily and you can always soften it by brushing through. Feel free to exaggerate a little if you want to bump up your brows.

- Follow through and fill in the whole brow, brushing upwards in light, quick motions – the light colour is subtle so it shouldn't look too much.

- Brush the powder through, focusing particularly on the starting point of the brows next to the nose – you want it to look soft. A harsh square where the brows begin looks weird and very unnatural.

STEP 2:

- Your brows are not naturally one shade. Like your hair, they contain hairs in several shades. The hair towards the bridge of your nose is also naturally sparser than the hair towards the outer edges of your brows, so you'll need a darker shade there to mimic the natural hair density.

- Take the darker shadow (on the same brush) through the outer half of your brow. If you feel that you need more definition along the underside of your brow, run the darker shade under the brow too and blend.

- Add more powder or brush the brows out as you prefer and feel free to set them with brow mascara if they get waggly.

- If you find that you've gone a bit wrong or would like a sharper finish, tidy the area with some liquid concealer on a flat brush.

And you're done – perfect eyebrows sorted.

CHAPTER 19

· LIPSTICK ·

There's something empowering about lipstick, particularly red lipstick. Regardless of your chosen colour, you make a statement just by wearing it. Lipstick is, like eye make-up, an expression of who you are. It has a transformative power. The perfect nude just makes you look effortlessly polished. A hot orange makes a room summery even in the depths of winter. A deep plum is sultry and subversive; it says 'Don't mess with me'.

Sometimes, we wear lipstick to express who we want to be. You might wear a bold red because you woke up brimming with confidence and you're in the mood to swagger about (which is a glorious sight to behold, so keep it up). Sometimes you need to make a statement, and sometimes you just want to have fun or express a good mood. Nothing in your make-up bag brightens and transforms a face quite so immediately as lipstick.

Finding your perfect lip colour

Red lipstick is in a category of its own, and to find the right shade of red, you should always be guided by the undertone of your skin (page 116). When it comes to the other shades though, you'll probably be both disappointed and bored to discover that your perfect lip colour is ... the colour of your own lips.

We know. Sorry.

But consider. When you see a photo of a celebrity and just adore their lipstick, you're not just admiring the shade of the lipstick. You're admiring the shade against their skin and what it's doing for them.

If you can achieve the same perfect marriage between your skin tone and a lipstick, it will be with a different shade, but the effect will be the same. You'll get the same glowing loveliness and perfect marriage of lipstick and skin tone, but the nude that looks great on Rihanna may be too dark a nude for you. Or the pale nude that looks radiant on Blake Lively might look like concealer lips on you, so choose carefully.

It's time that we as a nation of women accept that we don't have to change the way we are to be beautiful. So whether you have pale skin, a myriad of freckles, sallow skin or a darker complexion, accept that it's all lovely. Embellishing what you naturally have is the quickest, easiest and most fulfilling way to look and feel more beautiful.

So that's literally it. Your perfect everyday shade is the closest colour you can find to your own natural lip colour. Have a good look at your lips in the mirror. If your skin tone is cool or warm, the likelihood is that your lips are too.

Pale people generally have a pink undertone. If you are more olive-complexioned, then you likely have a browner or peachier undertone. Dark skins tend to have a slightly bluer undertone to lips.

If your lips are pinkish, then a pinkish shade will work better on you. If your lips have a slight blue undertone, then a brown- or pink-mauve hue will suit you best. If your lips have

It's time that we as a nation of women accept that we don't have to change the way we are to be beautiful. Embellishing what you naturally have is the quickest, easiest and most fulfilling way to look and feel more beautiful.

*Your perfect lip colour is
. . . the colour of your own lips.*

browner undertones, then a brown-based nude will look most natural.

Head into a department store (early in the morning is best, so that you can have the lipstick stand all to yourself before the other customers arrive) and hold the bullets up to your lips to see which is the closest match. When you think you've found it, swatch the shade on your hand to ensure that it is the colour it appears to be. For the love of all that's holy, don't swatch testers on your mouth. Because diseases.

Try to go for a moisturising formulation if this is going to be your everyday lip colour. That way it will feel nice to wear and the light reflection will give the illusion of more volume to the lips. And since the shade is matched to your lips, if it wears off throughout the day, you don't have to worry about a Pamela Anderson lip line waiting to scare the bejaysus out of you when you finally get a chance to look in the bathroom mirror.

To ensure the best possible staying power, apply your favourite lip balm, blot lips with a tissue and then apply your lipstick with a good quality lip brush. The brush works the product into the lips more than applying straight from the bullet will. Blot your lipstick and apply another layer. Blot again, and apply another layer. A nuclear blast won't get that lipstick off now.

Beauty decoded: Cupid's bow

Cupid's bow: The double-curved puckered area of skin just above the centre of the upper lip, which is believed to resemble Cupid's bow.

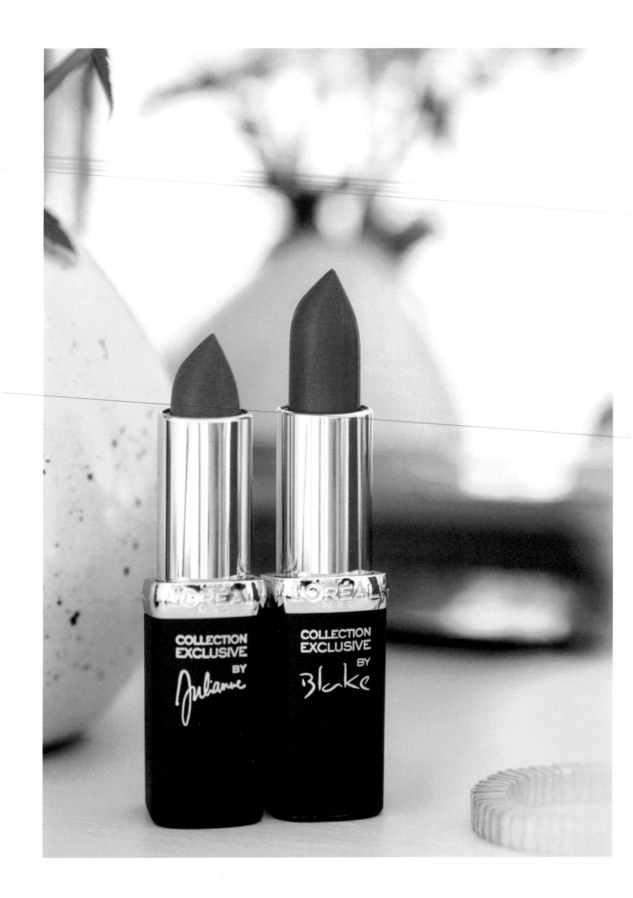

The best lipsticks

THE NUDES

For complexions with pink undertones, a pinkish nude is perfect. Chanel Rouge Coco Shine in Boy has a sheer moisturising formula and softly shiny finish. It's polished lips in a bullet. Tom Ford Lip Color in Blush Nude is suitably neutral and works for a wide range of skin tones. The buttery formula can't be beaten for opacity and smoothness.

Rimmel Apocalips Lip Lacquer in Nude Eclipse is a more traditional yellow-toned beige nude. It won't flatter pinker skin but on skin with yellow undertones, it enhances the natural warmth of the skin and is the perfect accompaniment to a smoky eye. The same goes for Charlotte Tilbury K.I.S.S.I.N.G. in Hepburn Honey. No concealer lips here. L'Oréal Color Riche Collection Exclusive in Doutzen's Nude is another great nude lipstick that pairs well with a strong smoky eye.

THE REDS

Many make-up lovers appreciate a good red. You just can't look scruffy in it, and a red lip is a make-up look all on its own. Anyone can wear it – it's just a matter of finding the right shade for your skin tone and the formulation that looks best on you. If your lips are on the thinner side, stick to a sheerer formulation, and try our lipstick application technique to cheat yourself a little more lip (page 222).

If your skin has a yellow undertone, warmer orangey red lipsticks like Nars Short Circuit will look fantastic on you. If you have a pink undertone or are on the pale end of the spectrum, colder blue-based reds like Mac's classic Russian Red will be right at home on your lips.

Chanel Rouge Allure Lip Colour in Incandescente is the perfect electric-orange red. It works wonderfully with all complexions from darkest to palest. Just make sure that you're feeling confident enough to wear it – this isn't one for the faint-hearted. But don't be too frightened of it – the matte texture takes the edge off the blast of colour and ensures that this classic shade will always be supremely chic.

Mac's Ruby Woo lipstick is the ultimate 1950s red and screams old Hollywood glamour. But beware: Ruby Woo's formulation is, for some reason, drier than that of all the other matte lipsticks from Mac, so make sure to prep your lips thoroughly and apply lots of balm beforehand. Once it's on though, only a good oil-based cleanser will get it off.

For a more moisturising formulation with a touch of subtly gorgeous sheen, opt for Rouge d'Armani Lipstick in No. 400, which is Giorgio Armani's iconic red shade. A sublime neutral red, it's not too hot or too cold. It's juuuust right. It smells like clean laundry, glides softly onto the lips and you need it in your life.

Box, named for Illamasqua chief, Alex Box, is a deeper, more dangerous red than classic '50s-inspired shades. It's not flat but softly light-reflective and daringly close to berry. A woman wearing this means business.

For an absolutely glorious affordable red, try Bourjois Rouge Edition Velvet in Hot Pepper. This matte liquid lipstick is true to its name. You'll have to look long and hard to find a hotter red. The formulation is excellent, so you don't have to bother with lip liner if you don't want to. It goes on thinly and dries down to a matte finish that miraculously doesn't feel drying on the lips. There's nothing sheer about it either. This is full-on, in-your-face red and it's effing gorgeous.

Beauty decoded: Lip liner

Lip liner has come majorly back into fashion since the rebirth of Kylie Jenner's lips. It can be used to add a little extra oomph to your lips, but it also gives lipstick something to grip and stops it from feathering out into the skin around the lips in that very unflattering way lipstick something does. Apply lip liner by tracing your cupid's bow and the centre of your bottom lip, and then joining up the edges. This is far less fiddly than trying to navigate your way around the lips. Then, fill in the lips before applying lipstick – this intensifies your lipstick colour and increases its lasting power.

THE DRAMATIC SHADES

A dramatic lip makes a statement of confidence and acts like an accessory to whatever you're wearing. Traditionally, red is the statement colour of choice, but it doesn't have to be. Earlier in the year, Illamasqua released a collection of blue lipsticks. You may not want to try a colour that's quite so unorthodox, but bold or unusual colours can look great and reinterpret a standard make-up look.

Mac Lipstick in Heroine is a blue-based bright purple that whitens teeth and looks beautiful with classic '50s make-up as an alternative to red. You need to be brave to wear it but once it's on, you'll immediately feel braver.

Bourjois Rouge Edition Velvet in Ping Pong is a brilliant bright fuchsia and is also Aisling's favourite. The liquid lipstick formula is somehow completely matte without being at all drying and its lasting power is so good that you don't need to bother with lip liner. This shocking pink livens up every tired complexion.

Nars Velvet Matte Lip Pencil is a wearable shade of orange that looks great on almost everyone. The shocking shade is a perfect contrast to for light or dark skin tones, and complements the warmth of anyone with yellow-undertoned skin in-between. Any very bright lipstick shade will draw attention to blemishes or discolouration elsewhere so make sure to conceal all diligently, and your lipstick will be the prime focus.

With darker skin that doesn't have pink undertones, bright pink lipsticks make a fantastic contrast. NYX Matte Lipstick in Shocking Pink looks amazing on darker skin tones, while Chanel Rouge Allure Lip Colour in Pirate is a fantastically pigmented shade that looks corally on dark skin and red on pale skin.

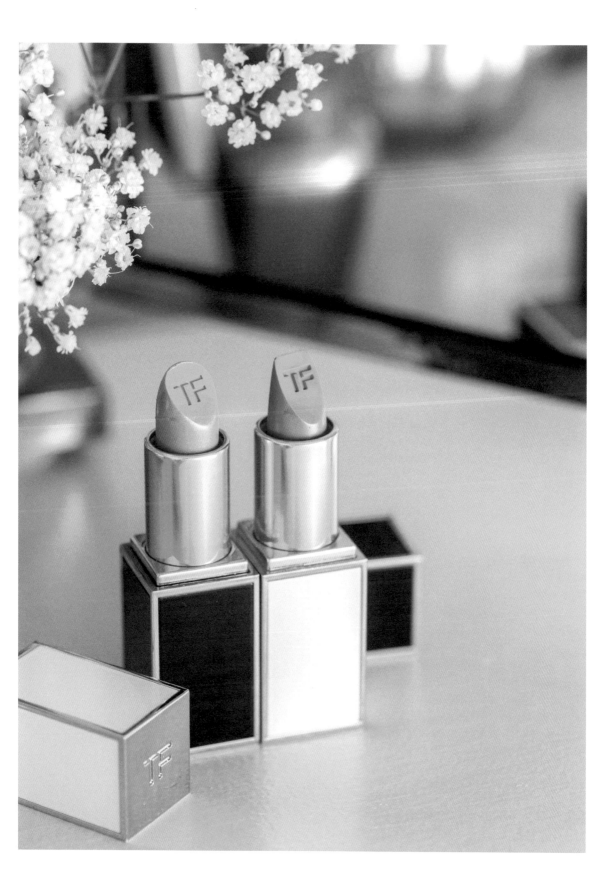

Beauty tutorial: Fake-the-feck-out-of-it lipstick

Finding the perfect nude lipstick can be a lifetime's work. Most of us go through a lot of duds (and money) in the search for the one. Once you've found it, there's still the small matter of applying it. Of course, you can just whack it on from the bullet and go about your business, but if you want to help one or both lips achieve a bit more volume, you'll need to put a couple of minutes' work in. What you'll get, though – fuller lips without having anyone stab you with things or massaging products loaded with cayenne pepper into them – is entirely worth the hassle.

Essentially, you need to overdraw the lips – but not like your Auntie Sally back in '87. No clown mouth here – you should be clever about it and overdraw only in certain places. We promise that when you're done, your lips will look like they're plumper and more evenly proportioned than they are. Lip liner is essential for this technique, so pick one up in a matching nude shade.

STEP 1:

- All lipstick looks best on prepared lips. Use a cotton bud to gently exfoliate. (You can also buy lip exfoliating products – or you can go to the press and get a little bit of sugar and rub that in instead. It will lift off all the gross peely skin and you'll be only gorgeous.) Then take your favourite lip balm (we love good old reliable Carmex) and buff it into the lips with a cotton bud to smooth away any crispy dry skin.

- Taking your liner, outline your cupid's bow and the centre of your bottom lip to begin with. This will ensure that your lips look even from the very beginning and it also ensures that we are not overdrawing in the centre of the lips, which is a dead giveaway and hearkens back to Pamela Anderson circa 1996, a place we never want to go. (So put down that brown lip liner. Bleugh.)

STEP 2:

- Follow the natural line of your lips, drawing out from the guideline you've made in the centre all the way to the outer edge of your lips.

- Colour your lips in completely with your lip liner; this gives lipstick something to grip and helps prevent it from bleeding. It also follows the layering philosophy – several thin layers ensure your lipstick will lasts through lunch and beyond. (Disclaimer: No lipstick immunity guaranteed through 3:00 am chilli cheese fries.)

- Now, you can start to embellish the natural lip shape a little with some very careful and subtle overdrawing. Take your time with this step, building on the line you've already created slowly and carefully. Don't fret about mistakes – a cotton bud dipped in eye make-up remover will solve any wandering liplines. Follow up with concealer on a lip brush, if you find that your foundation has become displaced.

- Try not to overdraw too much in the centre of the lip – you have lots of room to embellish on either side of the cupid's bow and to the left and right of the middle of the bottom lip.

- If your lips are disproportionate (if the top is bigger than the bottom or vice versa), embellish the lip that needs it and minimally line the other. The trick is to have a really good look at your lips. They're rarely identical on both sides of the cupid's bow, and few of us are lucky enough to have two evenly plump lips.

STEP 3:

- When you're happy with the lip shape you've created (you don't have to overdraw if you don't want to; sticking to your natural line is perfectly okay. Whatever makes you feel good), it's lipstick time, which we all know is the best bit.

- The best possible method of applying lipstick is to work several thin layers into the lips with a good lip brush. The brush should be small and soft with a very clean edge to keep lips looking sharp rather than blurry. You can apply it straight from the bullet but that way, you're not really working it into the lips. Particularly with intense colours like red, layering is essential or you'll end up with lip liner but no lipstick by the end of the day.

- Apply one layer of lipstick over the entire area, then blot on a tissue. Repeat once or twice for lipstick that will withstand quite a lot of abuse (and mayonnaise).

- Don't worry if your hand slips at this stage either. It's nothing to worry about. Just apply some concealer to a clean lip or eyeliner brush and clean up the edge again.

- Long-wear lipsticks last longest, but they can be a little drying on the lips. If you're wearing lipstick and eating, you will have to touch up a couple of times during the day or evening. But don't worry. This method will keep your lips in place and keep you looking chic all day long.

If you're scared or think that your lips are too thin for lipstick, try this method with a nude, coral or pink shade. You'll feel transformed.

The best possible method of applying lipstick is to work several thin layers into the lips with a good lip brush.

LIST OF PRODUCT IMAGES

P202
Lancôme Hypnôse Star Mascara

EYEBROWS
P209
A selection of eyebrow pencils and eyeliner
including:
Estée Lauder Double Wear Stay-in-Place Eye Pencil
Chanel Stylo Yeux Waterproof Long-Lasting
    Eyeliner
NYX Collection Noir Glossy Black Liner
Clinique Skinny Stick

LIPSTICK
P218
L'Oréal Color Riche Exclusive Reds
P221
Tom Ford Lip Colour
Tom Ford Lip Color Sheer

INDEX